DESIGNING HEALTHCARE SOLUTIONS
WITH MICROSOFT® BIZTALK SERVER 2004

PUBLISHED BY

Agility Press - An imprint of the Mann Publishing Group
208 Post Road, Suite 102
Greenland, NH 03840, USA
www.agilitypress.com
www.mannpublishing.com
+1 (603) 601-0325

Copyright © 2004 by Mann Publishing Group.

All rights reserved. No part of the contents of this book may be reproduced in any form or by any means without the written permission of the publisher. For questions about rights and permissions, send e-mail to permissions@mannpublishing.com.

ISBN: 1-932577-18-1
Library of Congress Control Number (LCCN): 2004115498
Printed and bound in the United States of America.
10 9 8 7 6 5 4 3 2 1

Trademarks

Mann Publishing, Mann Publishing Group, Agility Press, Rational Press, Inc.Press, Farmhouse Press, NetImpress, The Rational Guide To, Start to Finish Guide To, Rational Guides, ExecuGuide, AdminExpert, VertiGuide, From the Source, the Mann Publishing Group logo, the Agility Press logo, the Rational Press logo, the Inc.Press logo, The Content Company, Timely Business Books, Rational Guides for a Fast-Paced World, and Custom Corporate Publications are all trademarks or registered trademarks of Mann Publishing Incorporated.

All brand names, product names, and technologies presented in this book are trademarks or registered trademarks of their respective holders.

Disclaimer of Warranty

While the publisher and author(s) have taken care to ensure accuracy of the contents of this book, they make no representation or warranties with respect to the accuracy or completeness of the contents of this book and specifically disclaim any implied warranties or merchantability or fitness for a specific purpose. The advice, strategies, or steps contained herein may not be suitable for your situation. You should consult with a professional where appropriate before utilizing the advice, strategies, or steps contained herein. Neither the publisher nor author(s) shall be liable for any loss of profit or any other commercial damages, including but not limited to special, incidental, consequential, or other damages.

Credits

Authors:	Jim Casey, Elizabeth Redding
Technical Editor:	Jeff Wierer
Copy Editor:	Jeff Edman
Book Layout:	Molly Barnaby
Series Concept:	Anthony T. Mann
Cover Design:	Marcelo Paiva

All Mann Publishing Group books may be purchased at bulk discounts.

DESIGNING HEALTHCARE SOLUTIONS
WITH MICROSOFT® BIZTALK SERVER 2004

Jim Casey
Elizabeth Redding

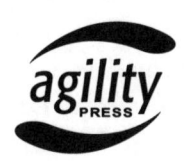

agility PRESS

An imprint of the mann™ PUBLISHING GROUP
www.mannpublishing.com

About the Authors

Since graduating from the University of Texas at Austin in 1997, Jim Casey has led the architecture and implementation of over twenty Fortune 1000 business integration projects utilizing a variety of technologies, including ERP, EAI, BPM, and service-oriented architectures. During this time, he has also played key roles in developing the strategy for industry solutions at several software companies. Jim is known for his ability to apply new technologies to real-world business challenges and is often a speaker at industry events. Jim currently lives in Dallas, Texas.

Elizabeth Redding is president and founder of Partner2Learn, Inc., a company focused on implementation services and training for business integration technologies. After earning her law degree from IIT Chicago-Kent School of Law in 1991, Elizabeth spent 6 years in private practice before entering the business integration field in 1998. She soon focused on the development of compliance strategies for mandated healthcare integration requirements.

Known for her domain expertise in healthcare as well as integration, Elizabeth has been instrumental in assisting medium to large healthcare companies, both payers and providers, with their business process integration strategies. As a Microsoft Certified Partner, her company, Partner2Learn, developed Microsoft's training materials on the BizTalk Accelerator for HL7. Partner2Learn continues to provide architectural, implementation, and training services for business integration and healthcare projects worldwide. Elizabeth currently lives in Chicago, Illinois.

Acknowledgments

This book would not have been possible if not for the hard work of many people. Special thanks to our publisher, Anthony Mann, for his patience and invaluable advice. We would also like to thank Jeff Wierer for his support of this project, ensuring the technical accuracy of the book, and for making the time to help us polish our message. Thanks goes to Jeff Edman for making sure we kept our deadlines and for doing a wonderful job of bringing clarity to the manuscript. Our gratitude goes to the many others who had a hand in making this book real, including Jan Shanahan, Mark Oswald, Kate Taneyhill, and Suren Machiraju. Last but not least, thanks to our spouses, Cathy and John, for letting us keep the light on a few extra hours at night and for their unwavering support.

Who Should Read This Book

This book is written for enterprise architects, developers, and consultants who are responsible for the design of medium-to-large scale software projects in the healthcare industry. We did not assume that readers would have a lot of experience working with business process integration platforms, or with BizTalk Server 2004, so this book should be accessible to the uninitiated in this type of technology. However, a good understanding of object-oriented concepts and general application programming experience is required to understand much of the content presented. The "Further Resources" section at the end of this book provides a list of resources that you can use to build your knowledge in these areas if you need a refresher.

Our goal in writing this book is to provide you with some insight into how to design systems using BizTalk Server 2004. With a flexible and powerful technology like BizTalk, proper design is often more critical to the success of the project than any other factor. As a result, we give you just enough "how-to" development information to understand the concepts. The focus of the book is on giving you an understanding of how the various components of BizTalk can be used *together* to build sustainable solutions, and why you would select one BizTalk component over another in your design.

We hope that you find the information presented in this text useful and welcome any thoughts or feedback you have about the ideas presented. To send feedback, visit www.agilitypress.com/feedback.

Jim Casey & Elizabeth Redding

November 2004

Conventions Used In This Book

The following conventions are used throughout this book:

- *Italics* — First introduction of a term.

- **Bold** — Exact name of an item or object that appears on the computer screen, such as menus, buttons, dropdown lists, or links.

- `Mono-spaced text` — Used to show a Web URL address, computer language code, or expressions as you must exactly type them.

- **Menu1➪Menu2** — Hierarchical Windows menus in the order you must select them.

- ➲ — Used to show a line of computer code or contents of a file that is supposed to be on a single line, but due to printing limitations in this book, the line is wrapped.

> **NOTE**
>
> This box gives you additional information to keep in mind as you read.

> **TIP**
>
> This box gives you additional technical advice about the option, procedure, or step being explained in the chapter.

> **CAUTION**
>
> This box alerts you to special considerations or additional advice.

> **BONUS**
>
> This box lists additional free materials or content available on the Web after you register your book at www.agilitypress.com.

Contents

PART I – Integration Planning 13

Chapter 1 – Overcoming Healthcare Integration Challenges 15
    The Price of Poorly Integrated Systems 15
    Information Technology Can Lead the Way 17
    An Alternative to Traditional Application Development 17
        Keeping Tabs on Operational Effectiveness 18
        The Integrated Enterprise 19
    Summary 20

Chapter 2 – Planning an Integration Strategy 21
    Why You Need an Integration Strategy 22
    Components of Enterprise Architecture 24
        The Plumbing: Infrastructure 25
        The Core: Business and Integration Logic 25
        The Building Blocks: Integration Patterns 25
        The Lynchpin: Integration Scenarios 26
        The Executive View: Enterprise Business Processes 27
    Elements of an Integration Strategy 27
        Inventory—What You Have 27
        Perspective—How You Look at Your System 28
            Bottom-Up 28
            Top-Down 30
        Usability 31
        The Team 32
    Summary 33

Chapter 3 – Adapters, Pipelines, Routing, & Server Configuration 35
Deployment and Configuration Tools 36
BizTalk Explorer 37
BizTalk Administration Console 37
Health and Activity Tracking (HAT) 38
Transport Handlers and Adapters 39
How to Use and Configure Adapters 41
Receive Locations 42
Receive Ports 42
Send Ports and Send Port Groups 42
Static vs. Dynamic Ports 43
Request-Response vs. One-Way Ports 44
Manually Creating a Send Port Bound to an Adapter 45
Global Variables for Adapters 47
Message Pipelines and the Message Box 49
How to Use and Configure Pipelines in BizTalk Server 52
Content-Based Routing 55
Summary 58

Chapter 4 – Metadata & Mapping 59
Metadata—The Blueprint for Information 59
Maps—Interpreting Data Between Different Systems 60
How to Use and Configure Metadata and Maps in BizTalk Server 2004 62
Creating Metadata 62
Promoted Properties and Distinguished Fields 68
Creating Maps 69
Configuring a Map for Runtime 74
Binding a Map to a Receive Port 76
Summary 78

Chapter 5 – Business Processes & Orchestration 79
Web Services—The Building Blocks of Orchestration..................... 79
Orchestration—The Foundation for Business Processes 81
When to Use Orchestration 84
How to Use and Configure Orchestrations in BizTalk 85
Creating Orchestrations 85
Configuring Orchestrations for Runtime.. 89
Advanced Orchestration Concepts 90
Correlation 90
Transaction and Compensation 91
Convoy 92
Summary 95

Chapter 6 – Business Activity Monitoring 97
What is a Business Activity? 98
BAM and Business Process Integration.. 98
A Framework for BAM 99
Data 99
Facts 99
Context 100
Dashboard 100
Business Activity Monitoring with BizTalk Server 2004 101
When to Use Business Activity Monitoring with BizTalk........................... 101
Building the BAM Definition 101
Building a Business Activity 102
Building a Business Activity Monitoring View 104
Deploying a BAM Definition File 110
Deployment Option 1: Real-Time Aggregation (RTA) 110
Deployment Option 2: OLAP Cube 111
Using the BAM Deployment Tool 112
Populating the BAM View and Tracking BAM Activities 114
Integration Using the BAM SDK 115
Integration at the Orchestration Layer with the Tracking Profile Editor............ 115
Aggregating Events with Continuation Tokens 120
Viewing BAM Activities 123
Charts and Graphs 124
Summary 125

PART II – HL7 and HIPAA 127

Chapter 7 – Integration Challenges of HL7 Processing 129

    HL7 Overview 130
        The HL7 Organization 133
        A Brief Look at the 2.x Message Structure 135
        Version 3, Anyone? 138
    Why Is HL7 Processing Special? 140
        A Look at a Sample Data Flow 141
        Integration Challenges 142
            Spaghetti, Anyone? 143
            Verified Delivery 143
            You Say MLP, I Say MLLP 144
            Real-Time? But We Save Resources by Batch Processing... 144
    Summary 145

Chapter 8 – The HL7 Accelerator for BizTalk Server 2004 147

    The HL7 Schema 148
    The BTAHL7 Receive Pipeline 151
        Working with the BTAHL7 Receive Pipeline 152
    The BTAHL7 Send Pipeline 155
        Working with the BTAHL7 Send Pipeline 155
    Working with the HL7 Schema in BizTalk 156
        Deploying the Project Containing MSH and ACK Schemas 157
        Deploying the Version-Specific Definitional Schemas 158
        Deploying Specific Message Schemas 158
    Configuring Acknowledgements 160
    Configuring Batch Processing 162
    Configuring the MLLP Adapter 163
    Mapping HL7 Data 164
    Summary 168

Chapter 9 – Integration Challenges of HIPAA 169

Rules that Affect the Healthcare Industry in the United States 170

Healthcare EDI 171

Affected Healthcare Transactions 172

Overview of HIPAA Standards 175

Required Transaction Sets 176

Introduction to the HIPAA Data Structure 177

Data Components 178

Elements 178

Segments 179

Transaction Sets 180

Control Data 183

All Together 185

HIPAA's Other Rules that Affect Integration 186

Privacy Rules 186

Security Rules 187

Summary 189

Chapter 10 – Using BizTalk Server 2004 for Your HIPAA Strategy 191

The Microsoft BizTalk Accelerator for HIPAA 3.0 192

Receiving Data Using the HIPAA EDI Adapter 193

Sending Data Using the HIPAA EDI Adapter 199

Importing Document Definitions 201

Configuring System Settings for the HIPAA EDI Adapter 202

Building HIPAA-Proscribed Security Measures 206

Summary 212

PART III– Extras 215

Appendix A – Fundamentals of Good Design 217
Have an Integration Strategy 217
Migrate Away From File-Based Integration 218
Use Smaller Transactions to Enable Better Business Visibility 220
Use Abstraction 220
Use Orchestration 221
Structure Projects to Have Multiple, Short Iterations 222
Apply Agile Software Development Techniques 223

Appendix B – HL7 Version 3 Processing with BizTalk Server 2004 225
What is HL7 Version 3? 225
Contents of Version 3 227
The Challenges of HL7 Version 3 Integration 229
BizTalk Server 2004 Meets the Challenge of V3 Integrations 230
Version 3 Integration Use Case: Establishing Interoperability between Version 3 and Version 2.4 Applications 231
    Integration Scenario One 232
        Configuring the HL7 Accelerator to Process the V2.4 Message 232
        Configuring BizTalk to Process the V3 Outgoing Message 237
    Integration Scenario Two 240
        Configuring BizTalk to Process the V3 Incoming Message 241
        Creating a Complete V2.4 Message Through an Orchestration 242
        Testing the Scenario 247
Summary 248

Glossary 249

Further Resources 253
Architecture and Strategy 253
BizTalk-Specific Resources 254
Business Resources 254
General Technology 254
Healthcare Resources 255

Book Registration 256

Part I

Integration Planning

Chapter 1

Overcoming Healthcare Integration Challenges

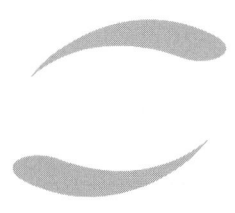

Electronic Health Records (EHR). Government mandates. Patient safety. Cost pressures. These are just a few of the challenges facing the healthcare industry today. In order to adequately address these issues, a different approach to building information technology (IT) driven solutions is needed.

Even though IT adoption in healthcare traditionally trails other industries, the challenges outlined above have reached a point of critical mass. We need to apply more sophisticated technologies to break through the barriers of operational inefficiency, poor visibility to information, and information latency.

The Price of Poorly Integrated Systems

Many of the challenges facing the healthcare industry today have their origins in an IT infrastructure that is predicated on building stand-alone applications to solve every problem. As a result of several decades spent following this approach, these applications have become thousands of individual "information silos." As the industry has become more collaborative, outsourced, and complex, these information silos have held us back.

For example, in a business process such as a patient diagnosis and treatment, multiple hospital departmental systems might be involved, the applications used by a third-party lab are also used, along with a practice management application used by the physician team, and the systems used by the insurance provider to process the claim. Unfortunately, much of the information sharing required in this process is paper-based, or poorly automated and easily broken. This results in lower patient care, increased patient risk, and higher overall costs.

This lack of integration manifests itself in many areas, including:

- **Electronic Health Records (EHR)** — Achieving a single, synchronized view of a patient's medical records will have tremendous benefits, including reduction in duplicate tests, reduced diagnosis errors, and significantly more accurate information available to front-line physicians and nurses. However, without integration among the systems of all of the parties involved, how will this ever be possible?

- **Cost pressures** — Properly integrated systems can enable more accurate and timely information to be provided at a significantly lower cost than currently available. These cost savings go beyond IT-oriented savings. For example, a business-level view of a process can identify bottlenecks and enable more efficient use of resources and improve execution. Without visibility into how work is being carried out, how do we know where to start with efforts to improve efficiency?

- **Government mandates** — Responding efficiently to mandates coming from external sources will continue to be a source of pain for many healthcare organizations. An agile infrastructure is required for the most efficient response. Implementing new applications without a plan of how they will work together will not lead to improved agility. How can we enable applications, both old and new, to be modified without breaking the links between other applications that rely on them for information?

Information Technology Can Lead the Way

The issues facing us are not necessarily new. Many of these challenges have been around for many years, and to be fair, certain aspects go far beyond information technology, such as politics, human nature, and organizing the many parties involved. However, there are some major pieces of the puzzle that can be solved using information technology.

In fact, by applying a few key technologies and a new approach to the problem, IT can help address many non-technical barriers to implementation, such as cost and flexibility of the system for end users. And by taking the initiative to overcome the challenges faced by IT, others involved in the process are more likely to make tangible progress.

An Alternative to Traditional Application Development

Unfortunately, for us to overcome the IT challenges we face as an industry, a different angle on the problem must be taken. A traditional approach just won't work.

What is a "traditional approach" and why won't it work? After all, IT has been doing pretty well over the past three or four decades, solving all sorts of business challenges and generally delivering spectacular return on investment (ROI). A traditional approach starts from the standpoint of building a single application to solve a business problem. For example, a financial application is the one place where all of the books are processed at the end of a fiscal period. An ordering system handles orders, and a lab system processes lab results. For many situations, traditional approaches such as these are the right way to go.

However, the traditional techniques of application development will not work by themselves for many situations today. This is because the root of many of the challenges facing the industry, such as EHR, is lack of integration of systems between providers, labs, and payers. There is no one application. The solution lies in the relationship between applications.

In areas where there is little or no integration, effective and timely patient care can be challenging. Consider the following excerpt from a healthcare industry organization:

"A study showed that within the U.S., 57 percent of patients had to tell the same story to multiple health professionals; 26 percent received conflicting information from different health professionals; 22 percent had duplicative tests ordered by different health professionals, and 25 percent of test results didn't reach the office in time for the patient's appointment."[1]

Unfortunately, a brute-force approach using traditional techniques will fail. For example, the Medical Records Institute (MRI) annually surveys over 750 healthcare professionals in the US and Canada. Since 2002, respondents have found "difficulty in finding an EHR solution that is not fragmented among vendors or IT platforms" to be one of the top 5 obstacles to implementing an EHR solution."[2]

Realistically, this type of problem does not lend itself well to being solved by one vendor. Rather, a more achievable and economical approach is to build a "virtual" or "composite" application based on parts of existing applications within each of the parties involved. Implementing EHR is only one aspect of the multiple healthcare challenges that can be solved with an integration-oriented approach.

Keeping Tabs on Operational Effectiveness

Not only will this new approach connect all the different applications together, but it will also give us insight into how effectively the different parties are interacting with each other in real-time.

Solutions built around an integration-oriented approach allow executives to answer questions such as:

- How long did the physician have to wait for radiology to produce needed x-rays?

- How often are patients asked to wait more than 15 minutes to be triaged?

- What areas of the hospital are experiencing the most volume?

- Can staff or beds be re-allocated to more effectively manage patient flow?

- Have the results of a previously-ordered test eliminated the need for additional tests at the lab?

- How can I process claims more efficiently across my subscribers?

- Are subscribers in my disease management program keeping to their treatment regimen?

This kind of contextual information about the process is crucial to the implementation of quality systems such as Six Sigma, which are gaining considerable traction in healthcare organizations. These programs aim to optimize processes, thereby reducing the number of errors and effectively managing human capital. However, without a solid foundation of facts provided by an integrated set of applications and third parties, such initiatives will have a difficult time providing meaningful and timely information.

The Integrated Enterprise

The elements required in order to build an infrastructure that can support this new approach are:

- A strategy for integrating the various people, data, and applications together across projects

- Alignment between end users and the chosen architecture

- A standards-based platform that can be used across a wide variety of projects to implement the strategy

- The ability to use industry standards such as HL7 and EDI

- Real-time monitoring at a business level to give executives new insight into the effectiveness of process improvement initiatives.

Microsoft BizTalk Server 2004 enables you to accomplish these goals by reducing the challenges associated with connecting diverse applications, and providing a platform to define and manage the business processes that are supported by those applications. The BizTalk Accelerator for HL7, an add-on component to BizTalk Server, allows you to rapidly build systems that communicate with each other using the HL7 2.x standard. The BizTalk Accelerator for HIPAA (Health Insurance Portability and Accountability Act of 1996) is also an add-on component that is focused on enabling communication between systems that must adhere to the HIPAA standard for electronic communication.

Each of these components will be discussed throughout the book. While every project and every organization is unique, many of the principles and best practices listed can be applied to most organizations. While a good amount of detail is given on how to build specific components of an integrated architecture, the focus of this book is on how these different pieces work together to create sustainable solutions over the long term.

Summary

Integration technologies can help the healthcare industry break through the barriers of operational inefficiency, poor visibility to information, and information latency that often result from a proliferation of "information silos." A true solution will require a non-traditional approach, rooted in all the elements of an integrated enterprise: an integration strategy, alignment between users and architecture, a standards-based platform, the ability to use industry standards, and real-time monitoring. As this book will show, Microsoft BizTalk Server 2004, with its support for HL7 and HIPAA, will enable you to reach these goals.

Chapter Notes

1. Robert Blendon, "Common Concerns Amid Diverse Systems: Healthcare Experiences In Five Countries," *Health Affairs* (May/June 2003), quoted in Markle Group, *Achieving Electronic Connectivity in Healthcare*, July 2004.

2. Medical Records Institute, *MRI Fifth Annual Survey of EHR Trends and Usage* (August 2003), http://www.medrecinst.com/pages/libArticle.asp?id=32.

Chapter 2

Planning an Integration Strategy

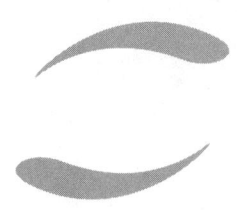

At the heart of any software application is an underlying approach to solving a business problem. Unfortunately, business problems are messy, and usually span multiple departments, processes, and even multiple businesses. On top of this, the many healthcare mergers and acquisitions that happened in the 90s brought together many formerly independent entities, each with its own unique application portfolio and processes.

These facts have left us with an array of technology pieces that have almost no way to share information with each other. The result? Solving problems in the real world involves tying together more than one application with the employees, customers, and suppliers that participate in a business process.

An integration strategy defines how various applications can be used together to solve a variety of challenges. This chapter will outline several approaches for building an integration strategy that will prepare your organization for a BizTalk implementation.

Why You Need an Integration Strategy

Have you ever seen how a custom motorcycle is built? First, you start out with a frame. Next, you buy an engine, some wheels, gas tank, and some other pieces. Through varying amounts of metal fabrication, welding, cursing, and sweat, all these parts come together and become your bike. Today's IT infrastructure goes through a similar process: a core set of financial applications usually form the frame, surrounded by a line of business applications and specialty applications, as seen in Figure 2.1.

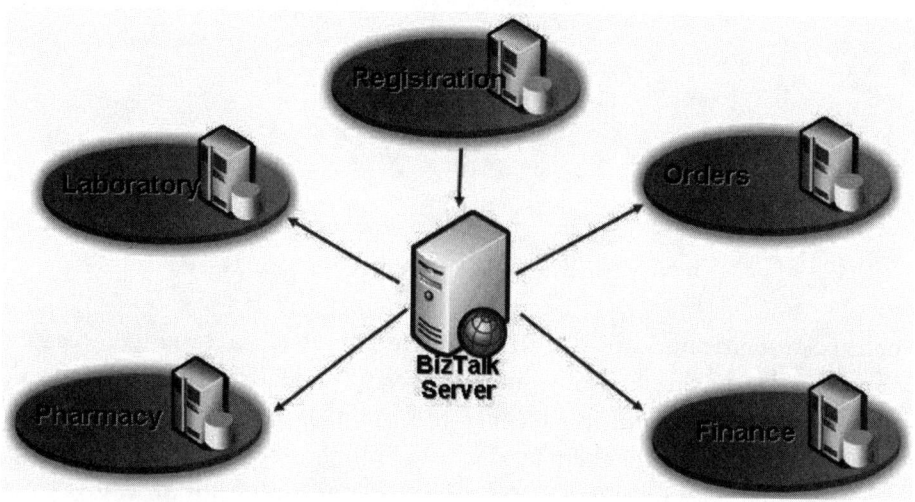

Figure 2.1: A Typical Landscape for a Healthcare Provider is Made Up of Many Applications.

The fact that the modern IT landscape is composed of lots of different parts from lots of different vendors is not an earth-shattering revelation. But, like a motorcycle, all these pieces must work together to become more than the sum of their parts. How the parts of your infrastructure come together is probably more important than what brand the parts are or the skill of the developer.

A critical piece of your IT strategy is determining how various applications and infrastructure will work together. An integration strategy is the mechanism through which you build a framework where relationships between business processes, applications, and infrastructure can be defined in a consistent and repeatable manner.

For example, the failure of many application implementations in areas like customer relationship management (CRM) indicates that even the best products are at the mercy of the quality of your integration strategy.

The ultimate goal of a software integration strategy is to have all of the various applications and infrastructure aligned in a way that enables you to:

- Improve the usability of information.

- Increase the business value of data. As initiatives such as HIPAA, electronic patient records, bar coding, and RFID play themselves out in the healthcare world, the amount of data is going to increase significantly. With the proper integration strategy, your organization will be able to act on these new information sources more easily, quickly, and effectively.

- Pick the best application for the job when buying new software. A solid integration strategy will enable you to focus on the business value an application brings, rather than worrying about whether or not it will work in your environment.

- Use technology assets. You can use applications and databases that you already own in new and powerful ways. However, working with existing applications doesn't mean that you have to miss out on new technology opportunities. An integration strategy will bring the tools, technologies, and training required to extend and enhance just about any existing system you have.

- More easily make changes to your applications. Like the human body, an IT landscape is always changing. A proper foundation of integration infrastructure is absolutely critical for building a change-tolerant system.

Components of Enterprise Architecture

Before you start building your integration strategy, you must first have a way to describe your systems and the way they interact in general terms. This foundation allows you to start to define some element or groups of elements in your enterprise and keep the terminology consistent. Most importantly, defining the major layers of your enterprise architecture helps to set the scope of work for integration projects by clearly articulating what each component needs to do and how it does it.

Figure 2.2 illustrates a useful way to describe an enterprise's IT assets for integration projects. There are five layers to any architecture:

- Infrastructure
- Business and Integration Logic
- Integration Pattern
- Integration Scenario
- Enterprise Business Process

Let's take a look at each of these layers in more detail.

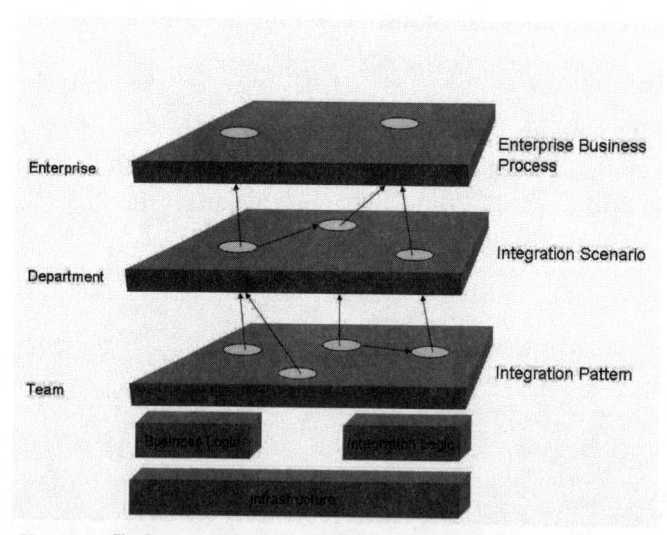

Figure 2.2: The Five Layers of an Enterprise Architecture and the Level in the Organization Where They Are Typically Managed.

The Plumbing: Infrastructure

The infrastructure layer is composed of the basic technical elements upon which everything else is built. If an IT environment were an aquarium, infrastructure would be the tank, water, and filter. Without these, the aquarium environment could not expand to support more complex components, such as fish.

Infrastructure typically consists of the operating system, application server (IIS), application frameworks (.NET or J2EE), messaging (MSMQ, JMS), portal framework (SharePoint or similar portal applications), database (SQL Server, Cloudscape), and directory server (Active Directory or similar).

The Core: Business and Integration Logic

Moving up a layer, business and integration logic lays out the heart and soul of the business. This layer contains the line of business applications and the logic that makes them tick.

While business logic is a term most people are familiar with, integration logic is often overlooked. *Integration logic* can be defined as those components responsible for managing the delivery, transformation, and routing of information as it flows between applications. The integration logic layer is the first layer where BizTalk Server comes into the picture.

The Building Blocks: Integration Patterns

The use of patterns for integration contexts has received a lot of attention recently. Basically, a *pattern* is a repeatable way to solve a reoccurring problem. Martin Fowler defines a pattern as "an idea that has been useful in one practical context and will probably be useful in another."[1]

Some examples of patterns include data access objects, facades, or even the best way to construct an array. Integration patterns might also include the best way to serialize messages, or the best practice for implementing a request/response interface.

Patterns are critical for building reusable components, such as web services. When consistently implemented across the enterprise, these integration patterns will manifest themselves as a layer of fine-grained services that can be used by both department and enterprise-level initiatives.

The Lynchpin: Integration Scenarios

As shown in Figure 2.3, an integration scenario is the interaction between the following components:

- **Business logic** — usually an application or set of applications

- **Integration logic** — how applications or services are connected to each other

- **Infrastructure** — the network, databases, hardware, and other components upon which business logic and integration logic run

An integration scenario is focused on the project/departmental level, and can be composed of integration patterns, business subprocesses, and microflows (workflows that do not encompass an entire business process). From a strategy-building perspective, integration scenarios allow you to identify gaps and look for opportunities to leverage existing components in your landscape.

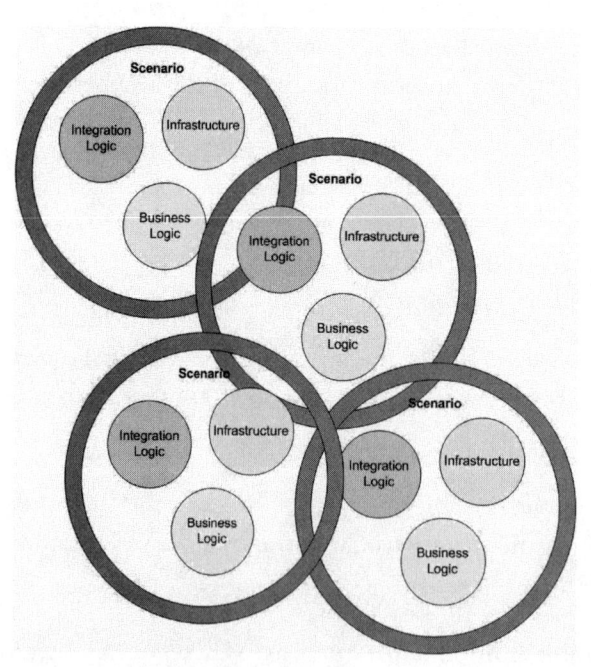

Figure 2.3: Elements of an Integration Scenario.

The Executive View: Enterprise Business Processes

At the top of the stack are the components that define cross-department, or cross-company, end-to-end business processes. Examples of an enterprise business process include how a hospital procures supplies for an emergency room, or how an insurance payer enrolls a new member. These are complex processes that span multiple applications, departments, and people.

The enterprise business process layer is often where the return on investment (ROI) is realized for projects. As a result, the temptation might be to skip the more technically-focused layers below and go straight to building the enterprise process. Unfortunately, this approach will usually result in an unsuccessful and unsustainable deployment.

In order to build an enterprise business process, all the layers below it (integration scenarios, patterns, logic, and infrastructure) must be properly aligned. The amount of complexity and the dynamic nature of business processes at this level are too great for a hard-wired or brute-force approach to be successful in the long run.

Elements of an Integration Strategy

So you have seen why an integration strategy is so important for the ideal deployment of the IT assets of the enterprise. Now let's explore how to get there. This section outlines the components of a successful strategy that will enable your vision.

Inventory—What You Have

Become familiar with your applications and infrastructure. You can significantly increase your agility and reuse with BizTalk projects by formally tracking and cataloging your existing business processes, metadata, applications, and interfaces.

When you look at how a typical integration project starts, you usually have a very tight completion time frame. Realistically, this is never going to change. However, by taking a snapshot of the existing IT landscape, you can prepare your organization for change, even though you may not yet have specific business requirements for your project. You can't be agile in the dark.

You probably already have an idea of your IT inventory, but it may not be readily accessible or up-to-date. Periodically update your inventory when major changes are taking place and place the information where the team can readily access it.

Perspective—How You Look at Your System

Once you have an accurate inventory, there are two basic ways you can look at it: bottom-up or top-down. Each view will tell you something different about your architecture, and give you the insight needed to design your scenario in the best way. Much like trying to solve a Rubik's Cube, it can be beneficial to look at your architecture from a couple different angles in order to arrive at a complete picture of the current situation.

Bottom-Up

This perspective starts with the smallest component in an integration scenario and builds upwards toward larger components. This view into your scenario is useful for understanding how fine-grained objects interact with each other on a project-by-project basis. Use this approach when making an inventory of your landscape in a particular area, when planning an upgrade of an application, and when you need to know what specific infrastructure components are required to support a project.

A pattern-based approach is a useful technique for describing how these smaller components interact. See the "Further Resources" section at the end of this book for resources for implementing pattern-based approaches to integration.

When to Use This View

A bottom-up approach works well to describe what already exists at the team level and sometimes at the departmental level. It can be a little difficult to use a bottom-up view as a starting point for a new project because you can easily end up with a case of "analysis paralysis" and losing focus on the business drivers for the project.

Given the detailed nature of a bottom-up view, you should restrict the scope to an integration pattern or an integration scenario. Think of this perspective as a snapshot of a small part of your architecture at a given moment in time.

While it might be tempting to build a single diagram that contains every detail of everything in your portfolio, often these drawings have too much information on them to be useful (see Figure 2.4). Furthermore, since a drawing of this magnitude takes a long time to put together, the information is often outdated.

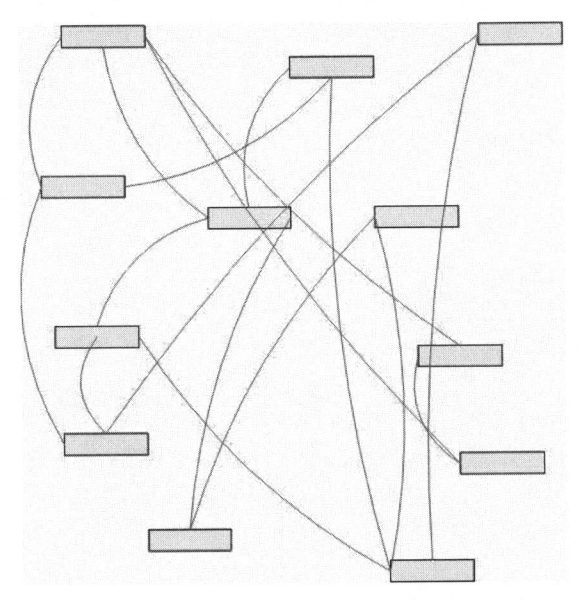

Figure 2.4: Spaghetti Diagram Resulting From Too Broad of a Scope in a Bottom-Up Diagram.

How to Build This View

Unified Modeling Language (UML) class diagrams, interaction diagrams, and Visio charts are all useful ways to view your architecture from a bottom-up perspective. While formal modeling techniques such as UML have tremendous value, sometimes an informal Visio can be just as effective.

Regardless of the technique you employ, a bottom-up view should include the following:

- Specify the technical names of all artifacts. For example, a method should be labeled with its actual name.

- List the interface that is called in participating applications. If it's a SQL statement, itemize the affected tables. If it's an API call, specify the method that is called.

- Illustrate the specific hardware involved, if necessary.

- Include what information is passed between artifacts, applications, and any participants. An arrow is not sufficient to show what information is being exchanged. If an Electronic Data Interchange (EDI) document is exchanged, put the transaction number above the arrow. If a method is called, what parameters are passed? What is returned?

Figure 2.5 shows an example of a bottom-up view.

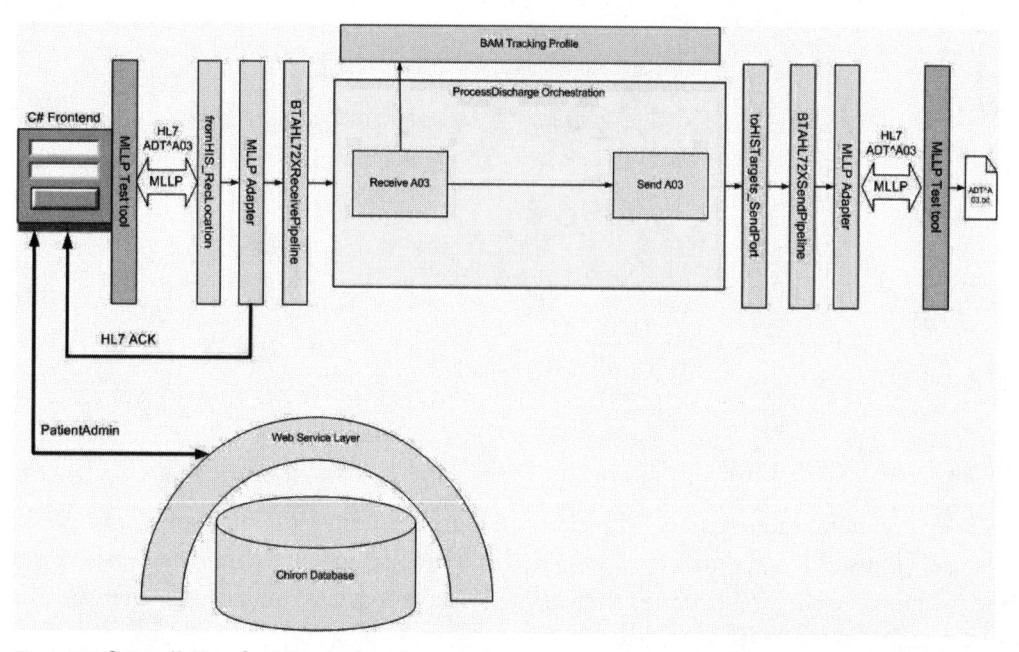

Figure 2.5: Bottom-Up View of an Integration Scenario.

Top-Down

At the opposite end of the spectrum is the top-down perspective. A good way to build a top-down view of your infrastructure is to use a business process management (BPM) approach. The idea behind BPM is to start by describing the key business processes in the business. For example, a payer has a certain way of processing a claim, and a hospital has a particular way of ordering medical supplies.

The concept of a business process is a well-established technique for describing how information technology assets and people work together in a specific business context. Howard Smith, co-founder of the Business Process Management Institute (at BPMI.org), defines a business process as "the coordination of end-to-end activities (manual, automated, usually both) that gets work done and provides value to customers."[2]

BPM is a concept that has been widely used and adopted by vendors, consultants, and industry analysts. As a result, you'll find a wide variety of terms to describe this approach. "Top-down" is an easily understood way of describing this class of tools, approaches, and methodologies without getting lost in the jungle of buzzwords.

When to Use This View

Top-down views based on BPM are the right approach to define an enterprise business process or a complex integration scenario. These layers typically require a relatively abstract view of what the business requires your IT environment to do. If you ever feel like you are losing touch with how your project is going to work in production, a process-oriented or top-down view will help you ground your technical requirements in the reality of the business need.

How to Build This View

Depending on the culture at your company, you may or may not want to have a highly formalized representation of your business processes. Many tools are available that can take a process model and generate the basic code structure required to execute that process. For example, the Orchestration Designer in BizTalk Server 2004 allows you to represent departmental business process flows during the design stage and easily add the necessary integration logic later. We will cover this topic in detail in Chapter 5.

Usability

Usability is often considered only important for developing user interfaces. But the user interface is only the surface of many interdependent components, each with their own features that make them more or less usable. As a result, the overall usability of a system is actually the aggregate of how well individual components that make up the system work together.

Even a less-than-optimal architecture will be a success if it's usable. On the other hand, superior technical execution is no guarantee of success. The best way to improve the usability of your architecture is to stay close to the users of the system.

Since most integration projects take place behind the scenes, it can sometimes be difficult to put a face to your user community. However, integration projects usually involve many applications, which bring along each application's users. As a result, integration projects have a larger user base than other applications in your landscape.

The Team

A vital element in your integration strategy is the team that executes your vision. The "Tragedy of the Commons" is a well-known anecdote about people looking out only for themselves. In this anecdote, ecologist Garret Hardin described several situations in which a society will destroy critical shared infrastructure if they think they can get a temporary short-term gain. Many IT landscapes can be viewed as common pastures that are abused by the people that rely on them most. While having complete control over your IT landscape is neither feasible nor desirable, some level of order must be brought to your environment in order to execute your integration strategy effectively.

To do this, you will most likely have to shift some organizational responsibilities. This change should result in the creation of a small team that will determine your integration assets and needs.

The integration team will enable the rest of your organization to execute their work in a way that maximizes reuse, increases overall maintainability of the landscape, and improves the collective knowledge in the organization about best practices for designing and deploying integration scenarios.

The integration team can accomplish this goal by:

- Taking a periodic snapshot of the applications, infrastructure, and integration logic that has been deployed

- Establishing standards for metadata, tools, and best practices

- Developing a knowledge base for integration techniques and patterns

- Mentoring departments who have integration projects underway

> **NOTE**
>
> As integration becomes more diverse, complex, and mission-critical, proper understanding of your IT portfolio is critical to future success. The establishment of an integration team will help integration projects evolve from a collection of fire drills to a coherent plan working towards a common vision for IT.

Summary

Have a plan before implementing your integration project with BizTalk. By examining your IT landscape from both a top-down and bottom-up perspective, you gain new insight into what design approach will work best. Through careful analysis of what you have already implemented, you can increase the agility of your team significantly. Finally, by taking into account the people involved—both the developers and the end users—you can make sure that what you build will be maintainable, workable, and usable to the business.

Chapter Notes

1. Fowler, Martin, *Analysis Patterns: Reusable Object Models* (Boston, MA: Addison-Wesley, 1997), xv.

2. Howard Smith, *Business Process Management 101* (July 2003), http://www.bmpi.org.

> **Did you know?**
>
> Joining the Microsoft Healthcare User Group (MS-HUG) is a great way to learn how to make your projects more successful and benefit from the experience of others in the field.
>
> You can learn more about MS-HUG at **www.mshug.org**.

Chapter 3

Adapters, Pipelines, Routing, & Server Configuration

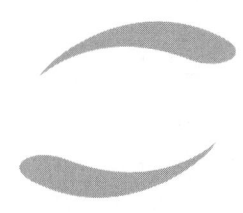

Regardless of your integration strategy, certain fundamental concepts are necessary to understand how to integrate your various processes, applications, and trading partners.

This chapter and the following chapters will introduce you to some basic integration approaches, and discuss how Microsoft BizTalk Server 2004 can be used as a platform for enterprise integration and business process automation. While we will get into some of the details, the focus is on understanding the basic concepts shown in Figure 3.1. It is assumed that you have access to a properly configured BizTalk Server 2004 instance.

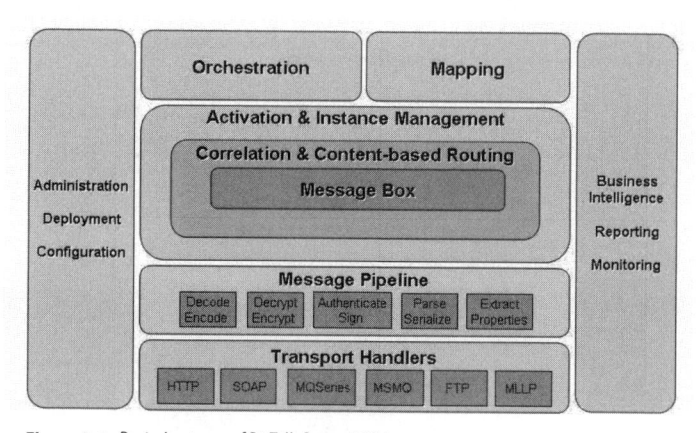

Figure 3.1: Basic Anatomy of BizTalk Server 2004.

Let's take a closer look at each of the layers in the stack. (Chapter 4 will discuss metadata and mapping; orchestrations are covered in Chapter 5 and business activity monitoring in Chapter 6).

> **NOTE**
>
> The ever-expanding list of acronyms associated with integrating software applications can be confusing. The Glossary lists common terms and acronyms relating to integration.

Deployment and Configuration Tools

After you've installed BizTalk Server, the first thing to understand is how to turn the server and its associated services on and off, and perform other basic administrative functions.

BizTalk Server 2004 comes with a number of tools for managing your infrastructure. These components are the "flight controls" of your BizTalk installation.

> **TIP**
>
> You can save a lot of time if you understand how to properly monitor your runtime environment. There are new monitoring and management enhancements in BizTalk Server 2004, such as Health and Activity Tracking, that can significantly aid your development process.

If you choose a "complete install" or "custom install" (and select **Development Tools** and **Monitoring Tools** during the install process), your system will be updated with new tools:

- BizTalk Explorer

- BizTalk Administration Console

- Health and Activity Tracking (HAT)

Chapter 3 - Adapters, Pipelines, Routing, & Server Configuration

BizTalk Explorer

This addition to Visual Studio .NET (shown in Figure 3.2) provides a way to manage BizTalk Server configuration and application settings. The look and feel of this tool is similar to the default Server Explorer provided by Visual Studio .NET. BizTalk Explorer allows you to manually define send and receive ports, start and stop orchestrations, and other configuration tasks. You can access BizTalk Explorer through Visual Studio .NET.

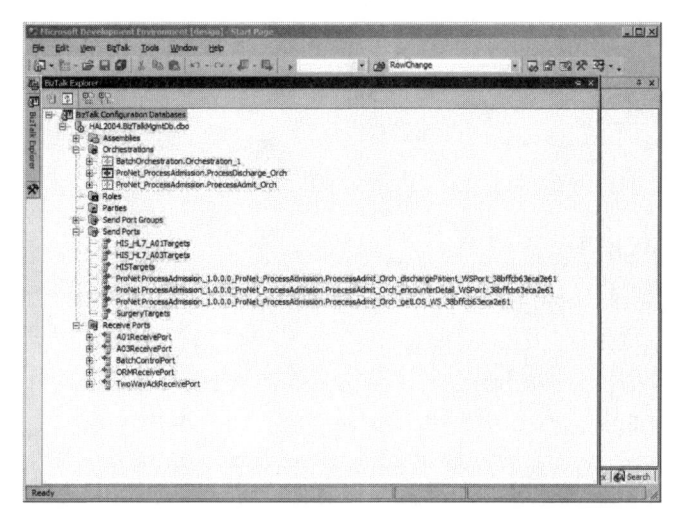

Figure 3.2: BizTalk Explorer.

Since BizTalk Explorer is only accessible through Visual Studio .NET, it is intended for use during development and testing. Usually, the people who monitor your system will not have Visual Studio .NET available to them. Because of this, the following tools do not require Visual Studio .NET, and are appropriate to install on machines that are responsible for monitoring the runtime production environment.

BizTalk Administration Console

The BizTalk Administration Console allows for basic monitoring and control of the server without the need for Visual Studio .NET. You can access this tool from the BizTalk Server program group on the **Start** menu. From the Administration Console, you can start and stop BizTalk Server instances, orchestrations, adapters, send ports and receive ports. The Administration Console is shown in Figure 3.3.

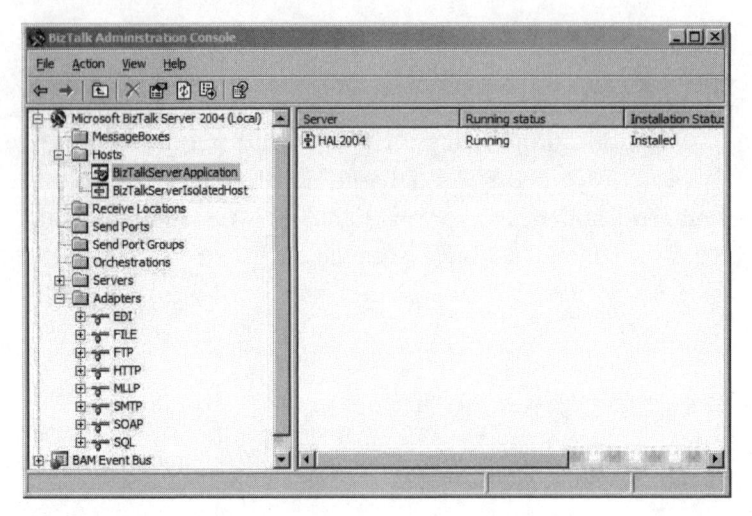

Figure 3.3: BizTalk Administration Console.

Health and Activity Tracking (HAT)

Health and Activity Tracking is new in BizTalk Server 2004 and replaces the older Document Tracking application provided in previous releases of BizTalk. Health and Activity Tracking allows a developer or administrator to monitor the technical details of messages as they flow through the system. HAT allows you to step through a running or suspended business process, inspect the data or metadata of a message, resume or terminate a service instance, or even set breakpoints in a process for debugging purposes. Using the database capabilities of SQL Server 2000, HAT gives you a number of ways to query processed messages along with the associated status of each message. You can access HAT from the BizTalk Server program group in the **Start** menu. An example of HAT is shown in Figure 3.4.

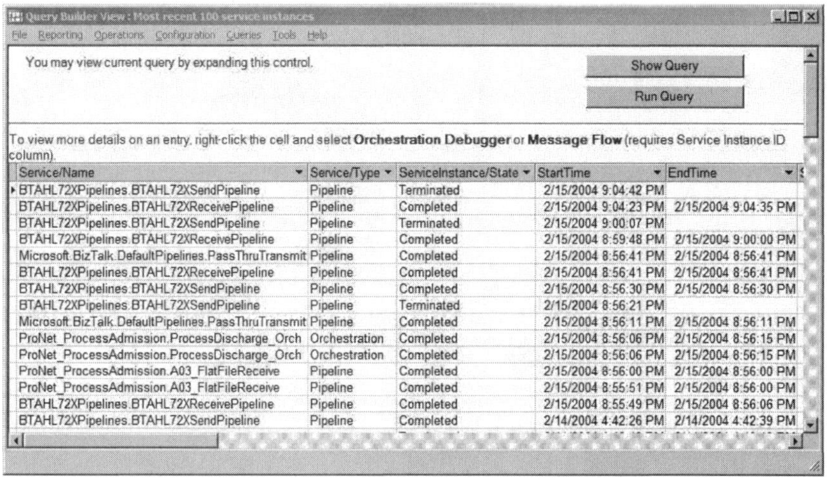

Figure 3.4: Health and Activity Tracking.

Transport Handlers and Adapters

At the bottom of the stack are the transport handlers, which enable the BizTalk Server to communicate with the outside world through standard protocols and application program interfaces, as shown in Figure 3.5.

Components in this layer have different names. Adapters, adaptors, transport handlers, connectors, and bridges, are all basically the same. Think of these components as providing the "dial tone" to a conversation between two software elements. Adapters range from the very simple (such as the ability to put a file into a directory) to the very complex (such as the ability to securely transmit HIPAA transactions over the Internet; for more on HIPAA, see Chapters 9 and 10). Until recently, you had to purchase adapters from the same vendor that you bought the other integration layers from (such as the messaging layer or transformation engine). However, most business integration platforms, including BizTalk, now support third-party adapters.

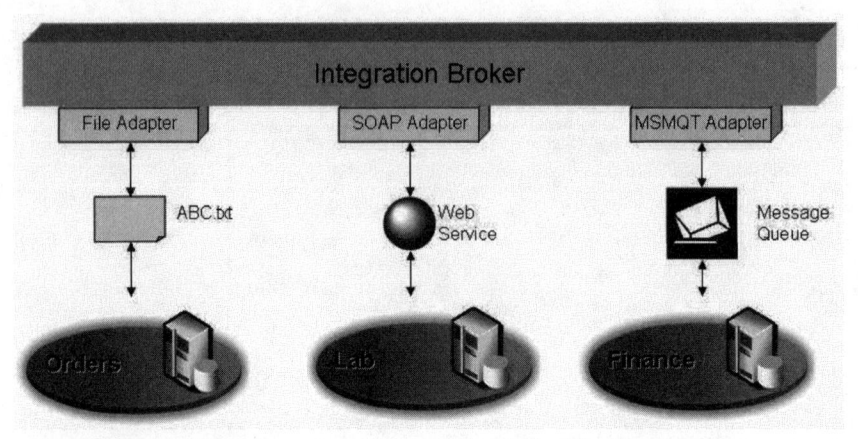

Figure 3.5: Adapters Allow the Integration Broker to Establish a "Dial Tone" With Other Applications.

Commonly-used adapters include:

- **File** — Gives you the ability to create a file in a specified directory.

- **HTTP (Hypertext Transport)** — Allows POST and GET commands.

- **SOAP (Simple Object Access Protocol)** — Gives you the ability to consume or provide a web service.

- **Database** — BizTalk includes an adapter for SQL Server)

- **MSMQ (Microsoft Message Queuing)**

- **MLLP (Minimum Lower Layer Protocol)**

- **FTP**

- **MQ Series**

Adapters are great because they allow developers to focus on building business logic instead of having to understand the details of a particular API or protocol. Because adapters are configured through a graphical user interface, they are relatively simple to set up and configure. Other benefits of this approach include:

- **Reduced complexity** — Most adapters support retry and rollback, so if the source or target for your integration scenario is unavailable or has some sort of problem, the integration infrastructure can handle the necessary rollbacks automatically.

- **Architectural integrity** — Adapters help enforce the best practice of separating business and integration logic from the transport details.

- **Easier to maintain and more robust** — A commercially-developed adapter for a particular application is more likely to be compatible with future versions of both your integration platform and the applications to which it connects, especially when working with commercial off-the-shelf (COTS) applications.

In short, adapters allow the integration project to roll out to production more quickly, and reduce the level of technical knowledge required to build an integration pattern, scenario, or business process. Adapters give you a much more sustainable and quality solution.

How to Use and Configure Adapters

There are a few additional BizTalk-specific concepts that you need to be familiar with when working with adapters:

- Send and Receive Ports

- Send Port Groups

- Receive Locations

All adapters in BizTalk are bound to a logical endpoint in the server. These endpoints are called *ports*, and provide features to enable architectural flexibility. For example, ports allow you to set up a business process even if you don't know how the message got to the process or how it is going to be sent.

Taking this concept a step further, grouping multiple receive locations together as a receive port allows you to use the same maps, pipelines, and orchestrations across multiple transports. For example, if a business process can receive data from either a file or MSMQ, you can use the same integration logic regardless how the message is delivered to BizTalk.

Receive Locations

In order for a message to flow into BizTalk, the server needs to know where to look and what to look for. A *receive location* holds the configuration information that tells the server which transport type to listen for, the location to look for messages, and what kind of message to expect. Basically, a receive location is where you select and configure an adapter. For example, to configure the file adapter to consume a file in a specific directory, you would create a receive location, bind it to the file adapter, and provide the directory location as part of the configuration of the receive location.

Receive Ports

Receive locations are logically grouped together as a *receive port*, which allows source systems to easily communicate with BizTalk using multiple protocols and transports. For example, if a lab application sends a nightly batch of information in a file, but sends rush orders throughout the day via MSMQ, you can create a single receive port for the lab application with two receive locations (one for a file, and another for MSMQ).

> **TIP**
>
> **If a source system sends information in more than one way, create a receive port with multiple receive locations for that system. This simplifies the configuration of the server, and encourages component reuse.**

Send Ports and Send Port Groups

Messages flowing out of BizTalk utilize *send ports*. Like a receive location, a send port holds the parameters used by the adapter at runtime for a particular interface. In addition, a send port can specify secondary transport options in case the primary transport is unavailable. Multiple send ports can be logically associated to each other through *send port groups*.

Chapter 3 - Adapters, Pipelines, Routing, & Server Configuration

A common source of confusion for newcomers to BizTalk is the difference between receive locations and receive ports, and send ports and send port groups. One easy way to remember the difference is that send ports and receive locations hold the adapter configuration. On the other hand, receive ports and send port groups are logical groups and do not hold any adapter-specific information.

In the example in Figure 3.6, BizTalk processes an inbound text file and sends it to the target via MSMQ, using adapters bound to a send port and receive location within the receive port.

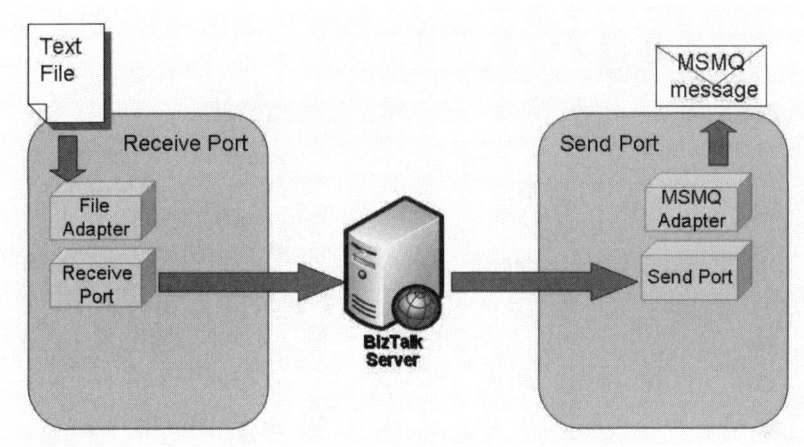

Figure 3.6: Adapters Bound to a Send Port and Receive Location Within the Receive Port.

Static vs. Dynamic Ports

Whenever you know that the source or destination will not change, and want a simple way to configure your environment, a *static port* can be used. This option essentially hard codes the URL for the source or destination.

Often, the actual destination for a message is not known until runtime. This situation is common when posting a message to an active server page with multiple arguments. *Dynamic ports* allow you to assign the physical location for a port at runtime. This can be done programmatically by setting the **Microsoft.XLANGs.BaseTypes.Address** property. Figure 3.7 shows this being set through an Expression shape in a BizTalk orchestration. (For more on orchestrations, see Chapter 5.)

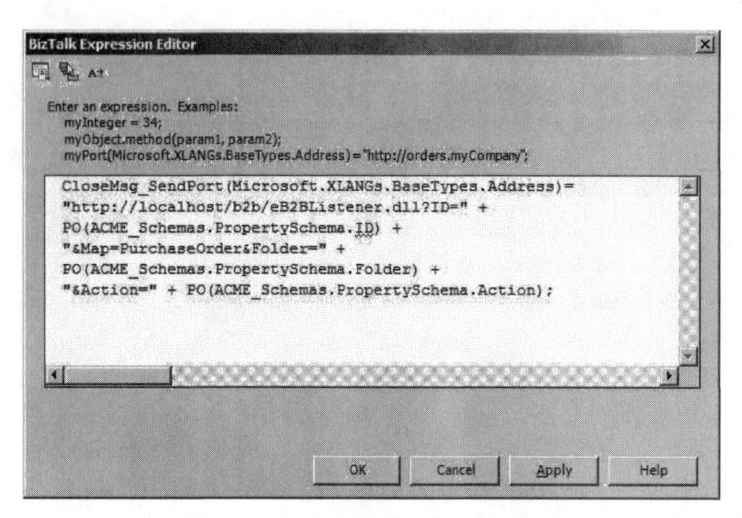

Figure 3.7: Setting the Address Property of a Send Port Through an Assign Shape as Part of an Orchestration.

Request-Response vs. One-Way Ports

Another architectural option available when creating a port is whether or not it is a *one-way* or *request-response* integration. A one-way port will behave in a "fire and forget" mode. Once the message has been sent successfully to the target, BizTalk will assume that any subsequent actions associated with that message will be handled by the target itself. For example, if a claim message is placed on an MSMQ queue in one-way mode, as soon as that message is placed in the queue, BizTalk will assume that the integration is complete. This mode is desirable when the protocol you want to implement does not support two-way communication.

If request-response is selected, the system will wait for an acknowledgement from the target application before BizTalk marks that integration as complete. Web services commonly use this technique. This mode is good for querying external systems and incorporating the response into an overall integration scenario. For example, if you want to validate a patient ID from an external system, you would use a request-response port to query the external system and determine how to proceed based on whether or not the patient ID query returned a positive or negative result.

Manually Creating a Send Port Bound to an Adapter

To manually create a send port bound to an adapter, a few simple steps are required.

1. From Visual Studio .NET, open BizTalk Explorer. Expand the configuration database for the server for which you want to create the port and select **Send Ports**. Select the port type. As discussed in the previous section, there are a number of different port configurations built into BizTalk, including static and dynamic one-way ports and static and dynamic request-response ports. For example, for a simple file-based interface, select **Static One-Way Port**, as illustrated in Figure 3.8.

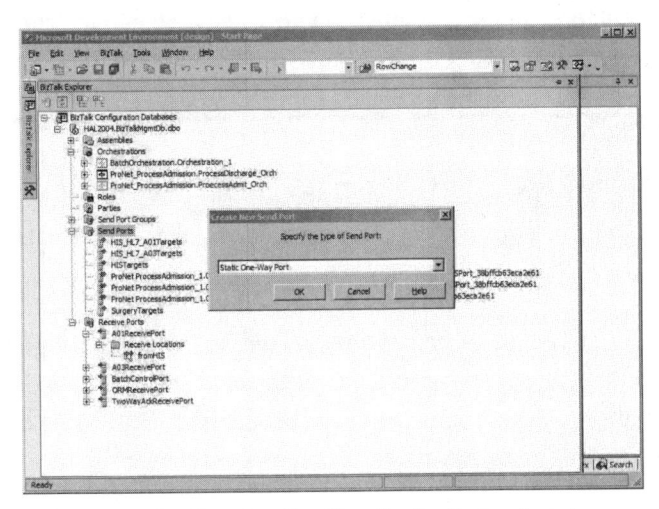

Figure 3.8: Specifying Type of Send Port After a New Port Has Been Created.

2. Select and configure the adapter you want to use. Adapters can be configured in BizTalk Explorer. One of the improvements in the 2004 version of BizTalk is that all development takes place in Visual Studio .NET. As a result, configuring adapters for BizTalk Server 2004 is straightforward, but remember to do your homework on the specific adapter you are working with. It is always well worth your time to read the documentation that comes with the adapter to make sure you are familiar with all of the functionality.

> **NOTE**
>
> What is the difference between an Adapter and an Accelerator? An Accelerator is an add-on product composed of BizTalk Artifacts that allow you to expedite or "accelerate" the process of solution development. An Accelerator may include: schemas, maps, pipeline components, orchestrations, application programming interfaces (API), new tools, user interfaces, sample code, additional documentation, or even new adapters. In short, Accelerators include pre-packaged functionality not already provided by the base platform. While some Accelerators are tied to certain industries (an example would be the BizTalk Accelerator for HL7 which is specific to healthcare; for more on the HL7 Accelerator, see Chapters 7 and 8), others may be built around standards applicable to a number of verticals, such as Electronic Data Interchange (EDI). Accelerators can be developed by Microsoft or third-party software providers.

What if there's no adapter available for your particular need? This occasionally happens, especially when dealing with a legacy application. If you find yourself in a situation such as this, you have three options:

- **Check for third-party adapters** — Microsoft created an "adapter program" so that third-party software vendors can create adapters. Several companies have built a library of over 250 adapters for BizTalk Server 2004. You can easily locate these adapters by browsing the BizTalk Server website at `www.microsoft.com`.

- **Build your own adapter** — Using the BizTalk Server Adapter Framework, Microsoft has made it possible for you to build your own custom adapter and have it accessible in BizTalk Explorer.

- **Wrap the application** — Build a service or component that will act as the middleman between the legacy application and the integration broker. While not an ideal solution, this approach has some benefits, including some level of abstraction and consistent interface design.

After selecting the adapter type, you will see a set of screens similar to Figure 3.9. For example, if you were to select the file adapter, this is where you would configure where the file is going to be put, whether to create a new file or append to an existing file, and what the file name is going to be. The name can be static, dynamic, or a combination of the two (e.g., myfile<message ID>.xml).

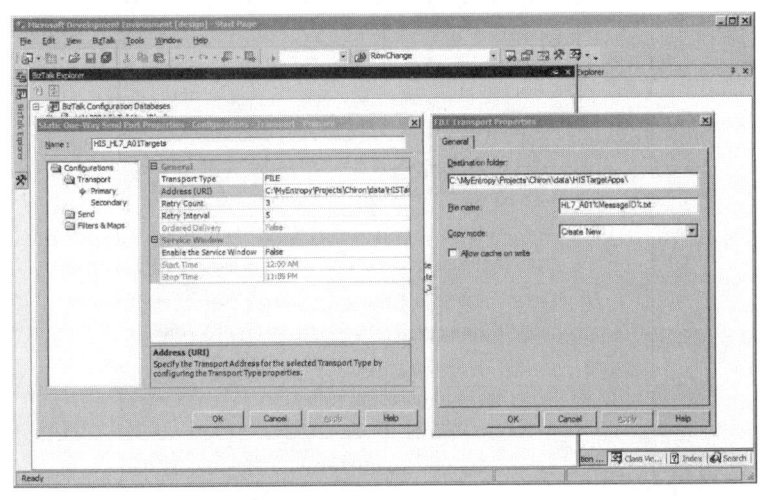

Figure 3.9: Configuring Adapters in the GUI.

Global Variables for Adapters

BizTalk has a built-in number of global variables that are available to adapters, such as Message ID. To reference one of these variables (actually they're macros), use %<variable name>% notation. Table 3.1 shows a list of the macros that can be used.

Macro Name	Substitute Value
%datetime%	Coordinated Universal Time (UTC) date time in the format YYYY-MM-DDThhmmss (for example, 1997-07-12T103508).
%datetime_bts2000%	UTC date time in the format YYYYMMDDhhmmsss, where sss means seconds and milliseconds (for example, 199707121035234 means 1997/07/12, 10:35:23 and 400 milliseconds).
%datetime.tz%	Local date time plus time zone from GMT in the format YYYY-MM-DDThhmmssTZD, (for example, 1997-07-12T103508+800).
%DestinationParty%	Name of the destination party. The value comes from the message context property BTS.DestinationParty.
%DestinationPartyID%	Identifier of the destination party (GUID). The value comes from the message context property BTS.DestinationPartyID
%DestinationPartyQualifier%	Qualifier of the destination party. The value comes from the message context property BTS.DestinationPartyQualifier
%MessageID%	Globally unique identifier (GUID) of the message in BizTalk Server. The value comes directly from the message context property BTS.MessageID.
%SourceFileName%	Name of the file from where the File adapter reads the message. The file name includes the extension and excludes the file path, such as foo.xml. When substituting this property, the File adapter extracts the file name from the absolute file path stored in the FILEReceivedFileName context property. If the context property does not have a value- for example, if message was received on an adapter other than File adapter- then the macro will not be substituted and will remain in the file name as is (for example, C:\Drop\%SourceFileName%).
%SourceParty%	Name of the source party from which the File adapter received the message.
%SourcePartyID%	Identifier of the source party (GUID). The value comes from the message context property BTS.SourcePartyID.
%SourcePartyQualifier%	Qualifier of the source party from which the File adapter received the message.
%time%	UTC time in the format hhmmss.
%time.tz%	Local time plus time zone from GMT in the format hhmmssTZD (for example, 124525+530).

Table 3.1: Global Variables for Adapters.

Message Pipelines and the Message Box

A message pipeline provides a series of discrete stages for processing inbound or outbound messages. These stages can include components for decoding/encoding, parsing/serializing, party resolution, or even custom validation. Pipelines are generally transport-agnostic and in most cases pipelines can be used with any adapter. There are two types of pipelines: *send* and *receive*.

A receive pipeline typically includes:

- A disassembly (DASM) component which parses incoming messages

- One or more components that validate the message against an XML schema (represented as an XSD)

- The configuration to make certain content in the message available as metadata in BizTalk variables

Send pipelines perform the opposite actions of receive pipelines, including:

- An assembly (ASM) component which assembles outgoing messages

- Validates the outgoing message against an XML schema (represented as an XSD)

- Makes certain content available globally as metadata in BizTalk variables

To summarize, message pipelines are either inbound (receive pipelines) or outbound (send pipelines), and are specified within a receive location or a send port. When a message is received from an adapter instance, the receive pipeline may perform actions such as disassembling the message, setting global attributes on that message (such as sender information, message ID, etc), and finally publishing the message as XML into a collection of SQL tables called the *message box*.

The message box is implemented as a SQL Server database, which is called BizTalkMsgBoxDb by default. You can view this database in Enterprise Manager just as you would any ordinary database. It is worthwhile to look at some of these tables to get a first-hand view of how BizTalk internal messaging works. It is critical to understand that you should never modify these tables or directly write or modify data in these tables. Doing so may irreversibly affect how BizTalk Server performs.

You can think of the message box as a location for a message to be momentarily held, allowing the system to drop off, pick up, or resume where a message left off in part of a larger business process. The message box also keeps track of who sent the message and where it was delivered, enabling an end-to-end audit trail which can be viewed using Health and Activity Tracking.

Keep in mind that orchestrations typically receive and send data through the use of ports. Orchestration design is covered in Chapter 5.

Once a subscription is activated, the message will pass through one or more send pipelines. The send pipeline reads the message instance from the message box, and may encrypt, assemble, or validate it if necessary. It then passes the message on to the adapter specified by the send port.

Figure 3.10 illustrates that send ports and receive locations specify which pipelines are used to handle messages published to or subscribed from the message box.

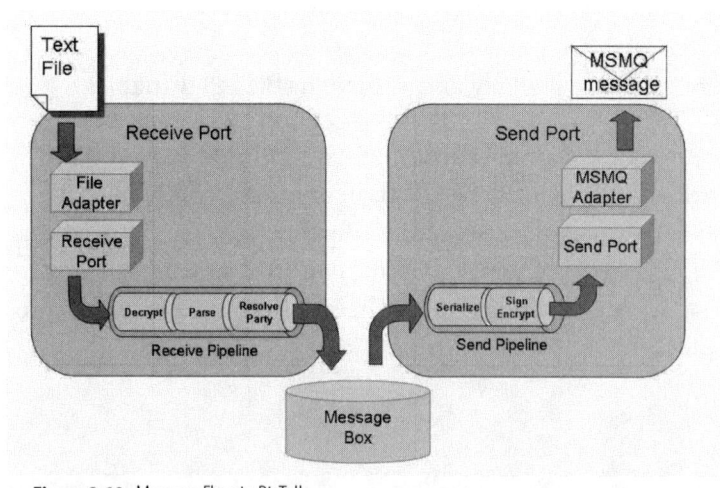

Figure 3.10: Message Flow in BizTalk.

BizTalk includes a couple of pre-built pipelines for use within your applications:

- **XMLReceive Pipeline** — Consumes well-formed XML. However, the content of the message is not available for routing or subscriptions (see the "Content-based Routing" section later in this chapter).

- **XMLTransmit Pipeline** — Constructs well-formed XML. Like the XMLReceive Pipeline, the payload of the message is not validated.

- **PassThruReceive Pipeline** — Accepts any message without parsing it. This pipeline is useful for initial testing or passing data, such as binaries, which do not require schema validation.

- **PassThruTransmit Pipeline** — Deserializes a message. Send ports that use this pipeline will receive the BizTalk internal XML representation of the message, not the original format of the message. This pipeline is useful for initial testing or passing data, such as binaries, which do not require schema validation.

Additionally, BizTalk ships with a number of reusable pipeline components for use with your custom pipelines. Some of these are:

- **Flat File Assembler** — Provides the framework to create non-XML documents. You associate this assembler with a pipeline you have defined using the pipeline editor in Visual Studio .NET (see the following section "How to Use and Configure Pipelines in BizTalk Server 2004" for details on how to do this).

- **Flat File Disassembler** — Provides the framework to parse non-XML documents.

- **Multipurpose Internet Mail Extensions (MIME) Decoder** — Typically used for parsing multipart messages as they are received by BizTalk.

- **MIME Encoder** — Typically used for assembling multipart messages as they are sent from BizTalk to message subscribers.

How to Use and Configure Pipelines in BizTalk Server

Let's assume you are not using one of the built-in pipelines and need to build a receive pipeline for an XML file you want to process. Use the following procedure:

1. Create a BizTalk project in Visual Studio .NET by selecting **File** ⇨ **New**. The new project will appear in Visual Studio Explorer. Right-click on the new project and select **Add a new item**. Select the receive pipeline option under **BizTalk Project Items** and click the **Open** button (see Figure 3.11).

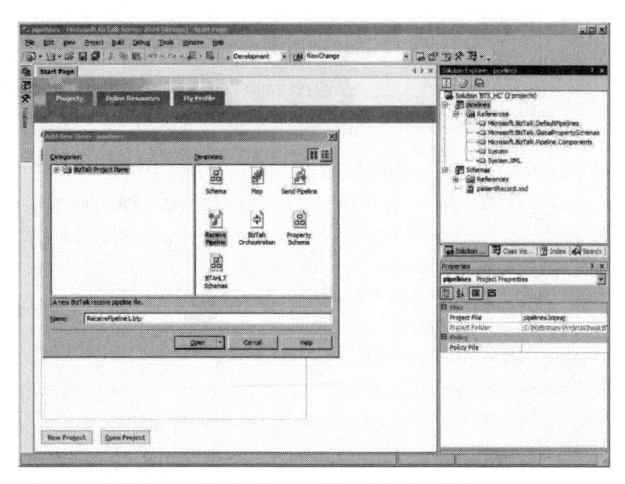

Figure 3.11: Creating a Receive Pipeline in Visual Studio .NET.

2. Define the pipeline. After you have added a new pipeline in the project, the pipeline editor will be displayed in Visual Studio .NET as shown in Figure 3.12. In this UI, you can define the behavior of your pipeline, such as what kind of messages it will receive, whether or not the message should be decrypted, which DASM to use, and any additional validation that is required. To configure the pipeline to receive a custom XML format, drag and drop the **XML disassembler** shape from the toolbox into the disassembler step in the pipeline editor.

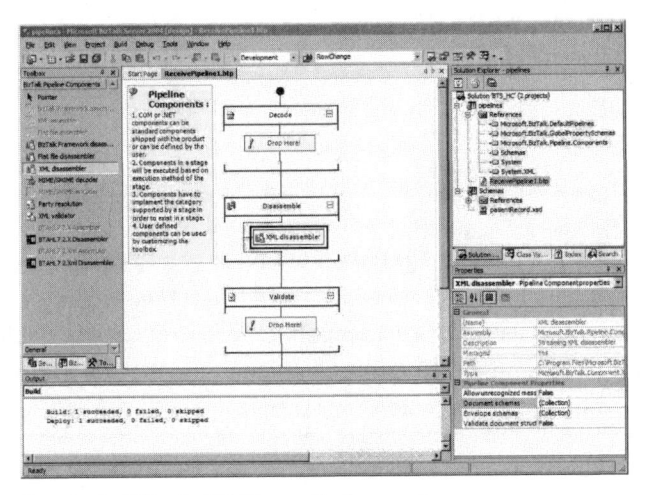

Figure 3.12: Adding the XML Disassembler Component.

3. Associate the schema definition for the file to the Disassembler shape. Under the **Document Schemas** property under the pipeline component properties window, click on the ellipses (…). You will see a screen similar to Figure 3.13. Add your schema definition and click the **OK** button (see Chapter 4 for information on how to create schemas in BizTalk).

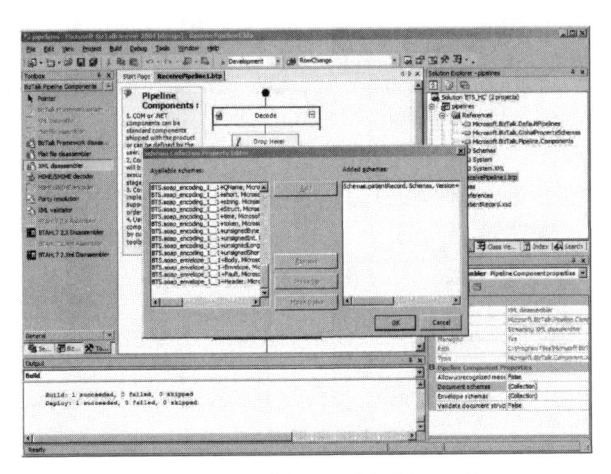

Figure 3.13: Associating an XML Schema with the Disassembler.

4. Build and deploy the project by right-clicking on the project and selecting **Deploy**.

> **NOTE**
>
> **When configuring BizTalk, remember that in order for you to be able to select a component (such as a schema contained in another project) and bind it to another component (such as a pipeline), you first have to deploy the project containing the referenced object. Refresh the BizTalk Explorer window, and you should be able to see your schema.**

> **TIP**
>
> **When assemblies are deployed to a BizTalk Server, they end up being published in the Windows Global Assembly Cache (GAC). To place an assembly (such as a BizTalk project) in the GAC, the assembly requires a strongly typed name. To give your project a strongly typed name, you need to generate a keyfile and associate that keyfile with your project. For information on how to do this, refer to the** *Deploying .NET Applications: Lifecycle Guide*, **available through Visual Studio .NET Help.**

5. Bind the pipeline to a receive location. In BizTalk Explorer, double-click on a receive location. This opens the receive location configuration dialog window, as shown in Figure 3.14. You will see a configuration entry for receive pipeline. Select this row and a dropdown list will appear. Select the pipeline you created. Fill out the remaining fields for the receive location and click the **OK** button. Once created, right-click the receive location icon in BizTalk Explorer and choose **Enable** from the pop-up menu. Once the receive location is enabled, your pipeline is activated and ready for processing.

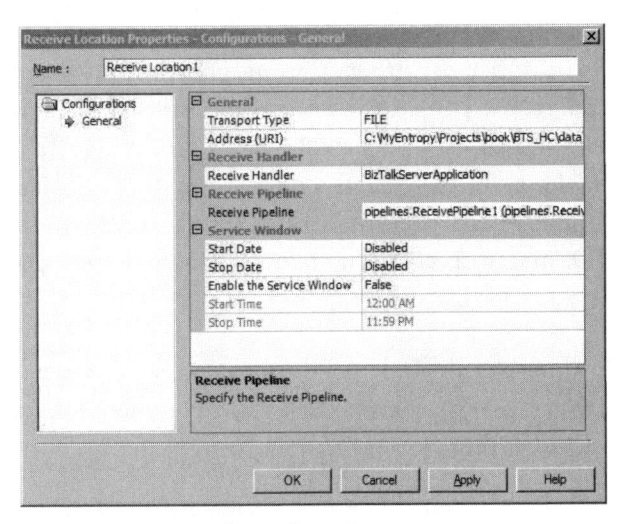

Figure 3.14: Binding a Pipeline to a Receive Location.

Content-Based Routing

So how does information flow through BizTalk Server? How are send ports invoked and send pipelines activated? With all the messages flowing through the system, how do you know what message is intended for whom? Content-based routing and correlation services provide the infrastructure that determines the path that an individual message or group of related messages will take through the system.

BizTalk accomplishes content-based routing through a publish and subscribe model commonly referred to as *pub/sub*. In this approach, the end point of every receive port is the "publication" of a document and its metadata into the message box. The starting point of any send port is a "subscription," which pulls data from the message box based on filter criteria.

The advantage of a pub/sub model is loose coupling between source and target systems. Under this model, source systems do not need to know who or how many systems are targets for a particular message. On the receiving end of the message, target systems can remain unaware of other targets, and unaware of the source system, allowing for highly flexible and dynamic message exchange.

It is important to note that BizTalk uses pub/sub internally, but can accept and send messages to and from queue-based systems, and connect synchronously with external systems where required.

Let's take a closer look at how pub/sub is implemented in BizTalk. When a message is processed by a receive port, a number of variables are populated that describe key elements about the message and become part of the process of publishing the message. Some of these variables are automatically set by BizTalk, such as **message ID**, receive port and pipeline name, etc. Others are defined at design time and associated with a particular message schema. These variables contain business data from the message payload itself, such as patient ID, diagnosis code, or claim number. These variables are known as *promoted properties*, and are discussed in Chapter 4.

Once the message has been consumed by BizTalk, we need to determine where to send it. The criteria for message delivery to a particular send port is called a *subscription*. A subscription can be either very complex or very simple, depending on your needs. Subscriptions can be:

- Based on technical information, such as the name of the receive port that processed the message

- Defined by specific values in the message payload being met

- Incorporated into any combination of business or technical data

A subscription is defined when a send port is created in BizTalk Explorer. To create or view a subscription for a send port, double-click the port and select **Filters and Maps**.

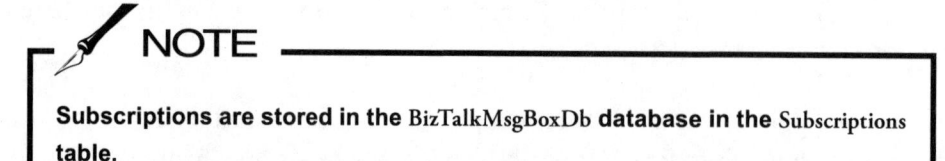

> **NOTE**
>
> **Subscriptions are stored in the** BizTalkMsgBoxDb **database in the** Subscriptions **table.**

In the **Filters & Maps** configuration screen (shown in Figure 3.15), you can define any number of criteria for your subscription. Properties that are available for applying subscription information against are listed in the **Value** column.

Under the **Group By** column, you can link multiple evaluation criteria together using the **and** grouping. Use the **or** grouping when any of the criteria must be true for you to receive the message on this port.

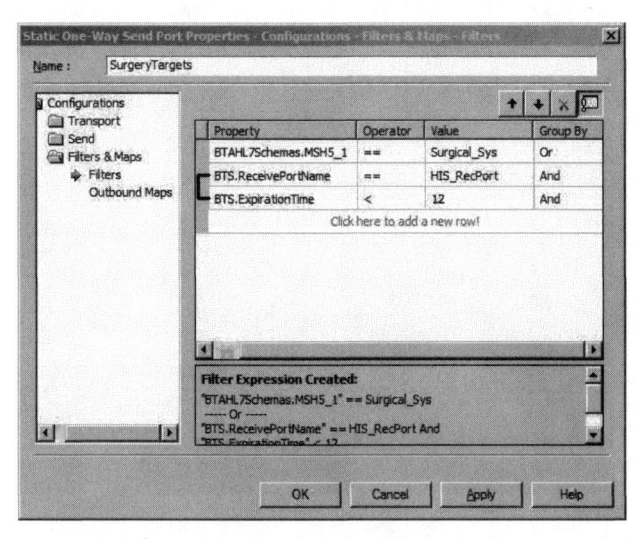

Figure 3.15: Defining a Subscription for the SurgeryTargets Send Port Using Multiple Criteria.

NOTE

If you don't see a message flowing through your send port, be sure you defined a subscription for it. The default for send ports is no subscription defined. If you don't define a subscription, you don't get any messages. Another useful tool for debugging is the subscription viewer utility. The subscription viewer can be found in the BizTalk installation directory.

Once you have completed defining a send port, you should always enlist and start it. This can be accomplished by right-clicking the send port and selecting **Enlist** and **Start**. Forgetting to enlist and start a send port is a common configuration error which can cause much confusion during debugging.

Summary

The nuts and bolts of BizTalk Server are important to understand, even if you're not going to be heavily involved with actual development with the product. After reading this chapter, you should have a grasp of adapters, send and receive ports, and send and receive pipelines. You should also know how the basic monitoring and configuration tools function. This understanding is essential if you are tasked with making the key design decisions for your integration infrastructure.

Chapter 4

Metadata & Mapping

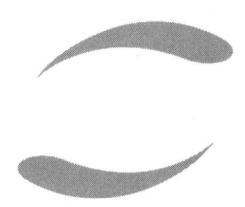

This chapter will explore how the BizTalk Schema Editor and Mapper can be applied to create and manage the various formats and semantics that are encountered when building an integration scenario. This chapter is intended to introduce you to basic schema and mapping concepts used in BizTalk Server 2004.

Metadata—The Blueprint for Information

Every application and system has its own unique way of defining data. For example, a hospital admission system will define the format of a patient's name differently from a Lab system. *Metadata* is the blueprint that defines how information is structured within a specific system or application. Database schemas, XML schema definitions, and Web Services Description Language (WSDL) documents are a few examples of metadata.

Metadata for a particular business message is constantly changing. In just about any project, business and technical requirements will include some addition or modification to the structure and content of data. As a result, the management of changes to metadata over time can be a difficult undertaking.

Even more troubling is that every system and application has its own set of metadata for a particular business process. When a process spans multiple applications, it is necessary to bridge the different schemas in a way that allows information to be understood by all applications in the process. A common oversight by project managers and architects is underestimating the amount of time and effort required to map various formats to each other.

The majority of integration costs are tied to the management of metadata and transformation between formats. One of the keys to the successful management of metadata in today's enterprise is the ability to rapidly and easily make changes. Graphical tools which include the ability to import metadata definitions such as database schemas and XML Schema Definitions (XSD) are critical to keep pace with the needs of end-users. In addition to these graphical tools, a code-free method of transforming and translating data from one format to another is required.

Maps—Interpreting Data Between Different Systems

Maps are the integration components that bridge the metadata of multiple applications at runtime. Figure 4.1 illustrates how maps and metadata work together to allow four systems to understand messages being sent between them. Maps enable this communication by performing the following tasks:

- **Transformation** — Changes the shape of the message from one format to another. An example of transformation is taking a legacy, comma-delimited file and turning it into a HIPAA-formatted claim. This task is sometimes shared with pipeline assemblers and disassemblers (such as converting a CSV into XML).

- **Translation** — Determines the equivalent value from an input field and assigns it to an output field. An example of translation is taking a patient ID of 1234 as input, and assigning the patient ID for the output to be ABCD. The translation here is to figure out that patient 1234 in system A is patient ABCD in system B.

- **Enrichment** — All of the data needed for the output is not present in the input message, so the map needs to populate the missing information from either business rules or logic embedded in the map. This might involve calling another system or service to gather the required information.

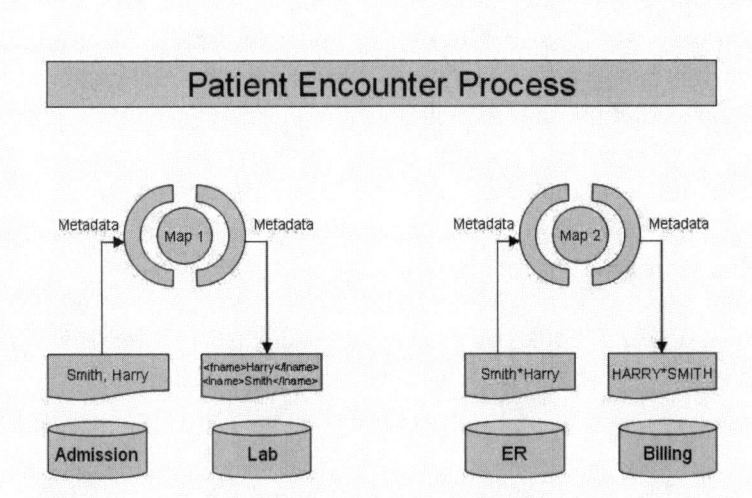

Figure 4.1: Maps Use Metadata Definitions to Bridge the Gap Between Various Formats and Semantics Associated with a Business Message.

In order for a map to perform these functions, it must have metadata properly defined. Well-defined metadata will make subsequent steps much simpler to execute, and is required before any mapping can be done.

> **TIP**
>
> If you find a map becoming too complex to manage, try redefining the metadata in a way that makes it easier to work with. For example, if you are parsing a very complex message, but you are only interested in the header, build a schema that only parses the header and puts the rest of the message into a large text field. This will make the map much easier to work with.

A question that often comes up when discussing mapping is "Why can't this just be coded in a standard programming language like C#?'

While manual coding can achieve the same end result, separating the mapping from the messaging layer and business process layers will give you a much cleaner architecture than if you were to lump mapping and application code together. For example, if you hardcode the mapping logic into the sending application, what happens when you add another application target? You have to modify your sending application to support the new format. Furthermore, what if the developer who created the code was replaced on a project and a new developer has to pick up the project? A graphical representation can be easier than reverse engineering code. The advantage of BizTalk in this circumstance is not the elimination of the need for transformation, but rather the elimination of the need to manage more code to do so. Since modifying applications is expensive, using a BizTalk map is a more economical approach.

Chapters 8 and 10 of this book cover metadata standards for the healthcare industry, but let's take a moment to cover some general design considerations.

How to Use and Configure Metadata and Maps in BizTalk Server 2004

There are several steps required to properly set up BizTalk to consume and create messages. In Chapter 3, we defined the configuration required to move messages and communicate with external systems. Now, we will define the message formats that will enable us to route messages based on the content of the message, also known as *content-based routing* (CBR), and transform and translate messages between formats (maps).

Creating Metadata

The first step to building a map is to determine your source and target formats. In the following basic example, your map will take a basic flat file and transform it to another format.

Let's say we have an input file that looks like the following: `1234, Casey, Jim, 100 Main Street, Dallas, TX, 75204, 214-555-5555`. The metadata defining this record layout is:

Patient IDPatient

Last NamePatient

First NamePatient

Middle Initial

Address Line 1

Address Line 2

City

State

Zip

Home

Phone

Even though this is a comma-separated value flat file, remember that as messages pass through the disassembler (DASM stage) of the flat-file pipeline, the data in the file will be parsed and represented within BizTalk as XML. Our output format is XML and is made up of these fields:

Patient

IDPatient

First Name

Patient Last Name

Home Phone

Address

City

State

Zip

Date processed

Based on the XSD schema created with the BizTalk Editor, the DASM will create an output file that looks like this:

```
<Patient First Name>Jim</Patient First Name>
<Patient Last Name>Casey</Patient Last Name>
<Home Phone>214-555-5555</Home Phone>
<Address>100 Main Street</Address>
<City>Dallas</City><State>TX</State>
<Zip>75244</Zip>

<Date Processed>01/01/04</Date Processed>
```

Use the following procedure to build the schemas.

1. In Visual Studio .NET, right-click on your BizTalk project and select **Add a New Item**. Choose **Schema** and name it `patientRecord` (see Figure 4.2). Click the **Open** button.

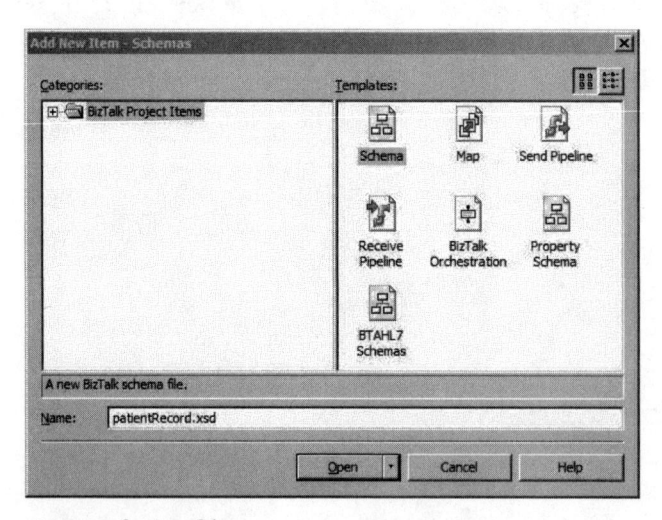

Figure 4.2: Creating a Schema.

Chapter 4 - Metadata & Mapping

> **TIP**
>
> A good strategy for organizing your XSDs is to keep related schemas together in their own project assembly. This keeps projects manageable and makes it easier to share schemas across multiple projects. If you know that a particular schema may be subject to frequent change, you may want to isolate that schema within a separate project. Remember that developing with BizTalk Server follows the general rules of .NET development. If you need to reference a schema located in a separate project or assembly, you can simply add a reference to your project.

2. Build the schema. The Schema Editor is a graphical environment where metadata can be defined and deployed to BizTalk. The editor is displayed after any schema is created, or when a schema is double-clicked in the Project Explorer. The Schema Editor will, by default, show two windows. A read-only XML representation of your schema is shown on the right, and an editable tree view is shown on the left. For the address schema, the first step is to rename the root node to be the same name as the schema file name. We now have a root element to which we can add child records or elements. These are represented as a tree structure in the left-hand pane, and as raw XSD in the right-hand pane. To add a schema element, right-click on the root node in the tree view and select **Insert Schema Node** and **Child Field Element**. After you have done this for each element in our example, the schema will look like Figure 4.3.

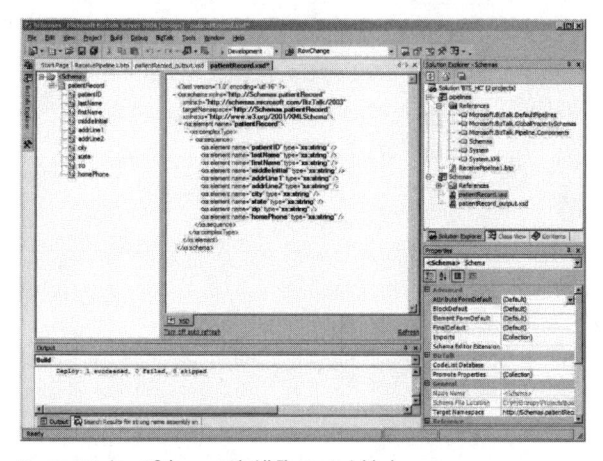

Figure 4.3: Input Schema with All Elements Added.

While you may be familiar with defining XML schemas to define XML data, we can use the Schema Editor to define both XML and non-XML data structures by using several extensions provided as part of the BizTalk platform. These extensions are found by clicking on the schema folder icon in the left-hand pane and then, in the lower-right property window, clicking on the ellipses next to the property for Schema Editor Extensions. For our example, select **Flat File Extensions** and click the **OK** button, as shown in Figure 4.4.

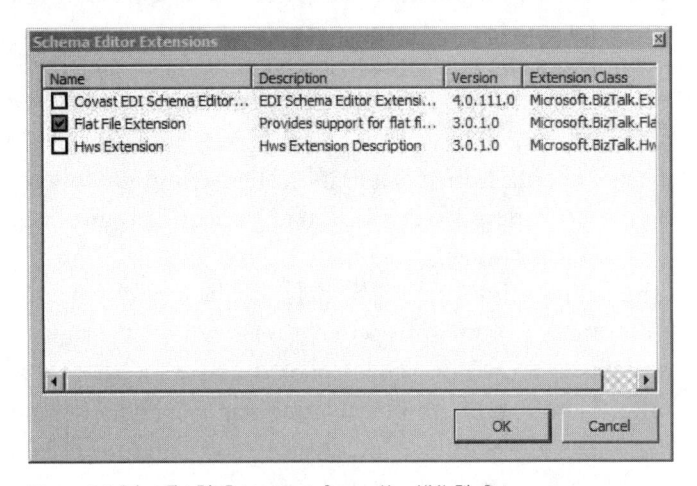

Figure 4.4: Select Flat File Extensions to Process Non-XML File Data.

3. Once the **Flat File Extension** has been selected, a new properties section will appear, allowing you to configure delimiters, terminators, and escape characters. To finish our example, select the root node (patientRecord). In the flat file properties for patientRecord, set the **Child Delimiter** to , (a comma), change **Child Delimiter Type** to character, and change the **Child Order** to Infix, as shown in Figure 4.5).

Chapter 4 - Metadata & Mapping

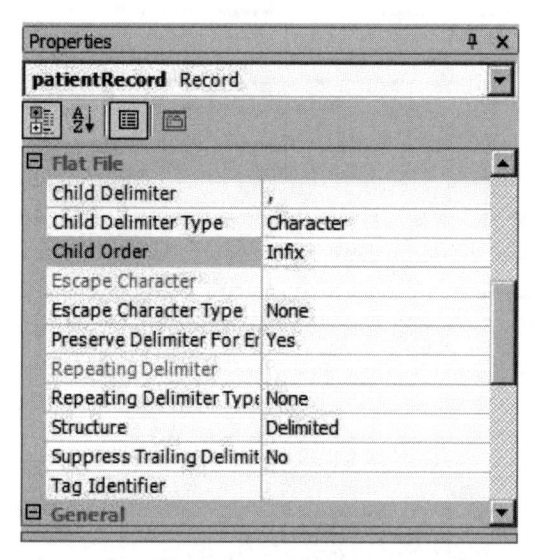

Figure 4.5: Setting Flat File Properties for the Root of the File.

4. Generate test data and validate the schema. You can generate test data for your schema by right-clicking on the schema in Solution Explorer (usually on the right-hand side of the Visual Studio .NET window) and selecting **Properties**. Figure 4.6 shows the window that will appear. This window allows you to define data to validate your schema definition against, or the file name for test data to be generated. Type in a file name and location for the test data to be placed and click the **OK** button.

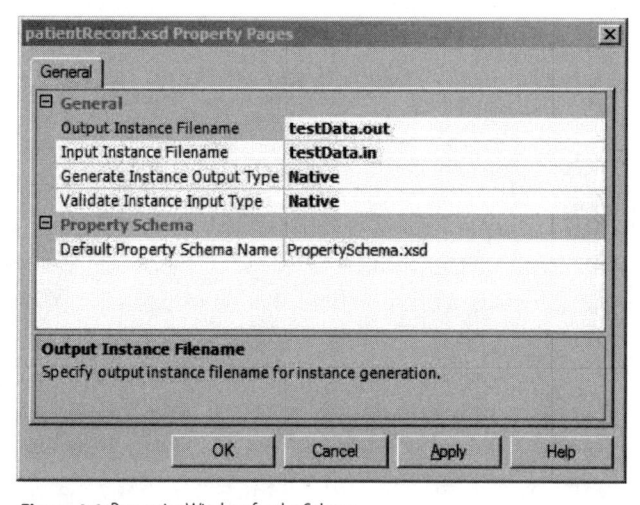

Figure 4.6: Properties Window for the Schema.

> **💡 TIP**
>
> **Waiting for valid test data can take a long time and is typically a big bottleneck on integration projects. Generating test data using the Schema Editor is a handy tool to keep developers busy. However, remember that nothing beats the real thing, so do not spend too much development effort before gathering actual test data to work with instead of the automatically generated test data from the Schema Editor. Conversely, if you already have an XSD, you can directly import it. If you have an XDR from a previous version of BTS, or a DTD, a conversion wizard is available with BizTalk that will turn these into XSDs.**

Promoted Properties and Distinguished Fields

By default, individual elements other than those that are part of a message context are not globally available to other components in the BizTalk runtime. When an element within the payload of a message is needed to determine subscription resolution (content-based routing), or for processing in an orchestration rule, you need to make that element globally available.

The process of making an element available to other components in the BizTalk environment can be done in one of two ways:

- Promoting the property

- Creating a distinguished field

Promoting a property creates a copy of the data held in that element in a globally accessible part of the message box. If, in our example, the state code of the patientRecord message determined which system would receive the message, we would need to promote the "state" element. An easy way to do this is to right-click on the **state** element and select **Quick Promotion**.

Once promoted, the content of the **state** element is mapped to a globally available schema, called a property schema (Property.xsd). The property schema is created in the same project as the source schema by default (don't delete it!), and once deployed, will make the **state** element available for subscription resolution and other actions.

The other way to make business data more visible in the process is to create a distinguished field. Promoted properties are good for things like send port filters, while distinguished fields perform better when trying to use a raw xpath query to access information within an orchestration. Also, distinguished fields allow you to access the data using dot notation within an Expression shape. For example, to access a field that has been designated as a distinguished field, you would enter `<message name>.<field name>`.

To create a distinguished field, right-click on the element you need and select **Show Promotions**. The dialog window shown in Figure 4.7 will appear. Make sure you are on the tab labeled **Distinguished Fields**, select the element you want and click the **Add** button.

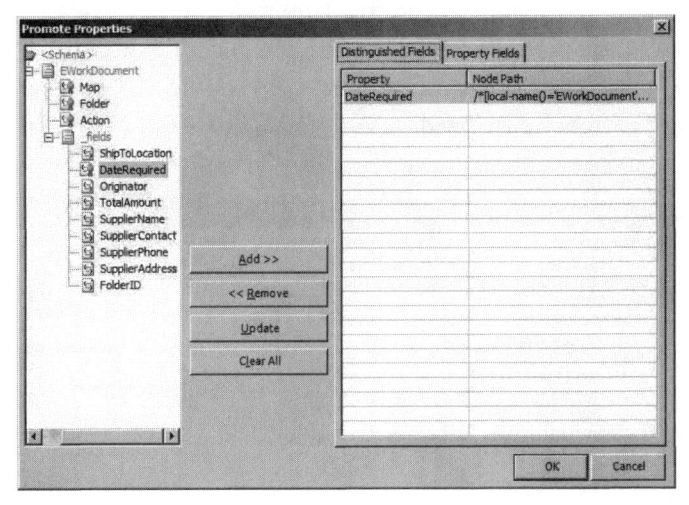

Figure 4.7: Creating a Distinguished Field.

Creating Maps

Once you have defined your input and output schemas, you are ready to create a map, according to the following steps.

1. Create a new BizTalk project to hold your maps and add a reference to the schemas project you created earlier.

2. Right-click the map project and add a new item. Select **BizTalk Map** under **BizTalk Project Items** and click the **OK** button.

> **NOTE**
>
> Consult Visual Studio .NET online Help for additional information on how to add a reference to an existing project.

3. After you click the **OK** button in Step 2, the BizTalk Mapper will appear inside of Visual Studio .NET. The Mapper is a graphically driven tool that allows you to visually define transformation, translation and enrichment for your messages. The map editor has two panes. On the left are the source schemas; on the right are the target schemas. To build your map, click on the link named **Open Source Schema** in the left-hand side of the Mapper. In the BizTalk Type Picker (shown in Figure 4.8), select your input schema, in this case **patientRecord.xsd**.

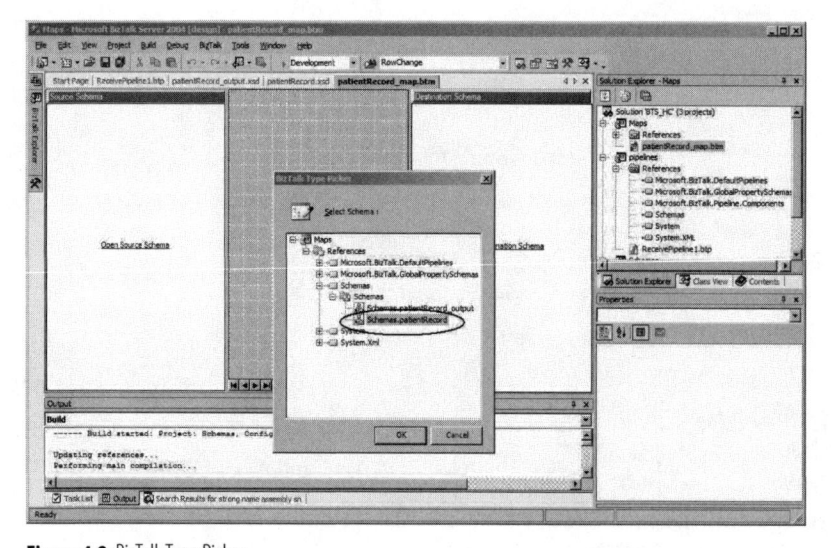

Figure 4.8: BizTalk Type Picker.

Chapter 4 - Metadata & Mapping

4. Each of these input/output panes is bound to a schema that you have defined or imported into a BizTalk project. For our example, click on the **Open Destination Schema** link on the right-hand side of the Mapper and select the target format (**patientRecord_output.xsd**). Figure 4.9 shows what the map will look like after a source and target schema have been selected.

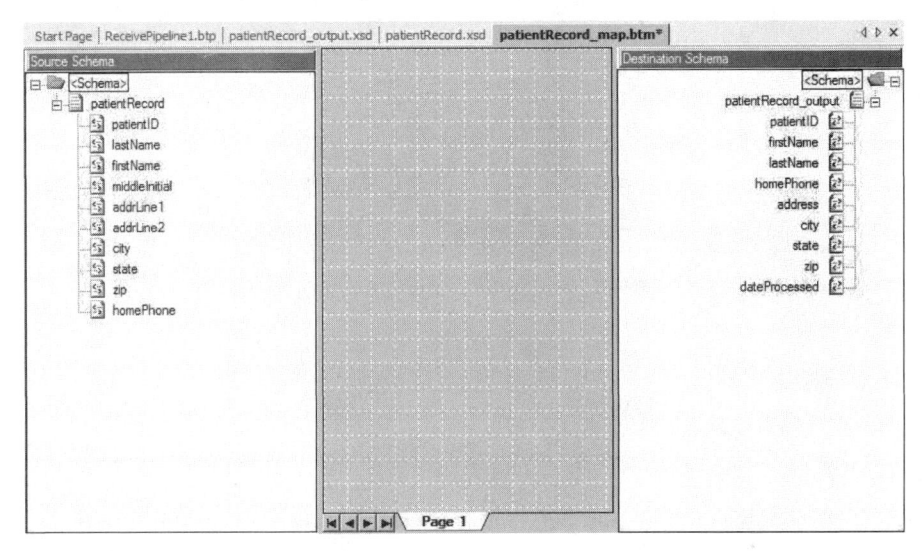

Figure 4.9: Source and Target Schemas After They Have Been Selected in the Type Picker.

5. Once we have bound an input schema and an output schema to the editor, we can begin mapping the input format to the target (see Figure 4.10). Defining the transformation rules is relatively simple. If you want to set the value of one field to be the same in the output, drag and drop the source element to the target element. For example, the values for the patient's first and last name are going to be the same in our target format as they are in the source, so all we need to do is drag and drop these elements to the corresponding elements in the target.

71

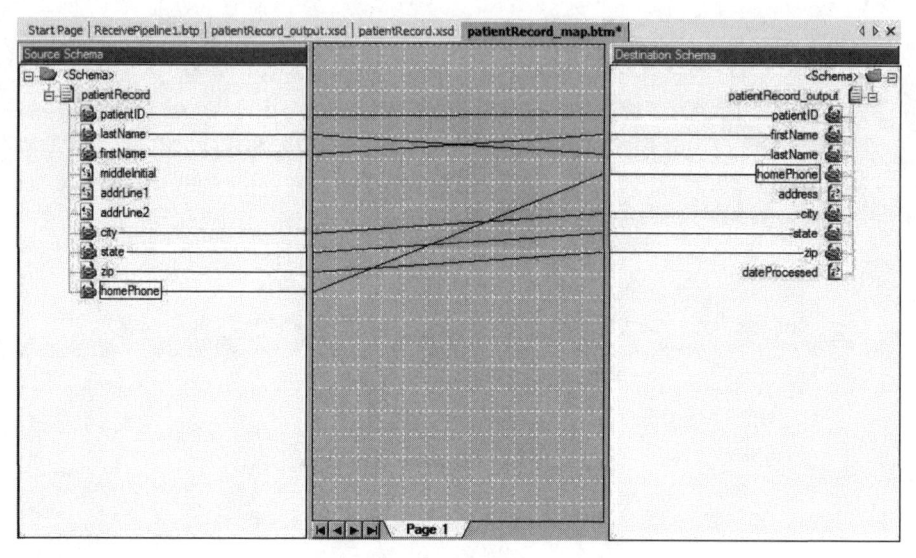

Figure 4.10: Dragging and Dropping Source Elements to their Corresponding Target Elements.

> **TIP**
>
> When a map (a .btm file) is created for BizTalk, it is actually made up of three parts: the input schema, the output schema, and an XML Stylesheet Language – Transformation (XSLT) file. This means that programmers who are familiar with other transformation tools should be able to pick up this part of BizTalk very quickly. Basing the transformation on an industry standard like XSLT also aids in migration from third-party mapping tools, if they adhere to the XSLT standard. If you have an existing XSLT, you can actually set a property on the map and skip the graphical mapping part altogether. Next, we'll look at functoids, where you can also use in-line XSLT as part of your map.

It would be nice if we could directly map fields to each other between documents. In the real world, this usually doesn't happen. With the exception of the simplest maps, you'll use functions such as string manipulation, math formulas, boolean logic, database access, and others, which can be inserted into the map grid between the source and target panes (see Figure 4.11). The BizTalk Mapper provides a toolbox of these types of functions. In BizTalk terms, these functions are referred to as *functoids*. For example, to concatenate the **addrLine1** and **addrLine2** elements and place the result in the target element named **address**, go to the toolbox and drag and drop the **string concatenate** object (under **string functoids**) onto the grid. Drag and drop both the **addrLine1** and **addrLine2** elements to the red box representing the concatenate functoid. Next, drag and drop the functoid object to the **address** element on the target schema. Now, **addrLine1** and **addrLine2** will be concatenated and placed into the **address** element in our output.

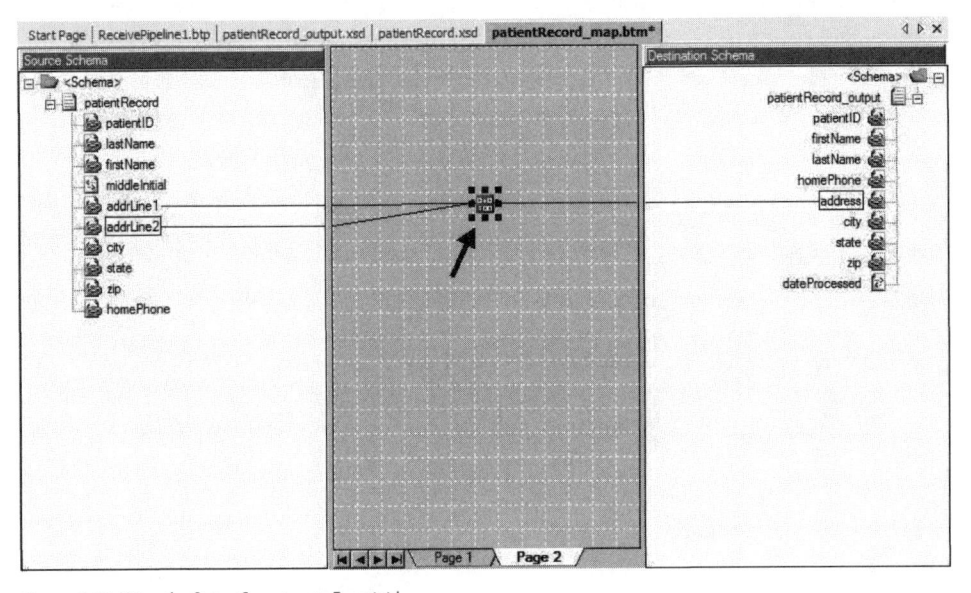

Figure 4.11: Using the String Concatenate Functoid.

TIP

Complex data structures can make the user interface of the Mapper difficult to read and maintain. To manage the complexity of maps, you should consider creating additional grid pages much like pages in an Excel workbook. Figure 4.11 shows an example of this technique (notice the Page tabs at the bottom center of the screenshot). Moving some mapping logic to another page can dramatically improve the maintainability of your maps. You can create additional Page tabs by right-clicking on an existing tab and selecting Add Page. Remember that the use of pages is for presentation only, and does not affect processing of your map rules.

Functoids offer a level of extensibility that XSLT can not provide alone. If you were to look at the XSLT behind the maps, you can see where BizTalk automatically extends the base functionality of XSLT to accommodate these functoids. If you are considering reusing the XSLT in other applications, keep in mind that these functiods are not supported outside of BizTalk. It is also worth noting that functiods can be chained so that the output of one functoid can be the input to another. Finally, if you cannot locate a functoid that meets your specific needs, you can always revert to the ever useful script functoid. The script functoid is an open-ended functoid that will allow you to write in-line code in C#, Visual Basic .NET, J# or even XSLT. Script functoids can also call code from referenced assemblies.

Once you have applied all of your mapping rules, you can test your work by right-clicking on the map object in the Solutions Explorer and selecting **Test map**. If everything worked okay, deploy the project.

Configuring a Map for Runtime

Once the project containing a map has been deployed to the server, it can be invoked in three ways:

- Being bound to a receive port

- Being bound to a send port

- From an orchestration through the Transform shape

The simplest way to run a map is to bind it to either a send or receive port, as shown in Figure 4.12. The steps and menus are essentially the same for setting up a send or receive port, and configuration can be completed very quickly.

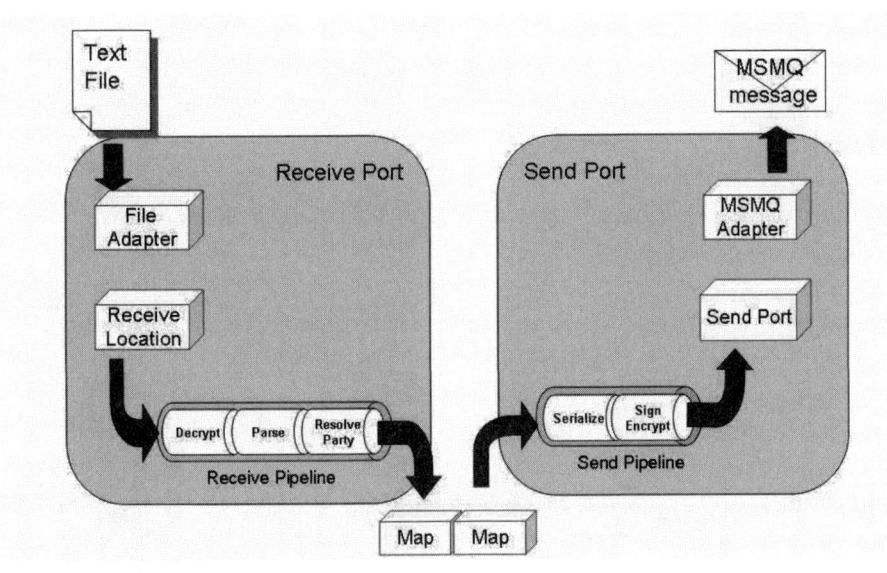

Figure 4.12: Binding a Map to Send and Receive Ports.

If your integration scenario or business process has no orchestration defined for it, bind your map to either a send or receive port. Even if you plan to use the map in an orchestration, usually it is a good idea to test out your maps using the simplest server configuration, and then add complexity (such as orchestration) later.

While setup is easy to configure, there are some subtle but important design decisions that will dictate where to bind your maps (send port, receive port, or orchestration).

If you choose to bind a map to the receive port, messages will be stored in the message box as the output format of the map. Therefore, any targets subscribing to that message will pick up the output of the map, not the original sending system's format. Use this approach when:

- Most targets require the message to be translated or enriched in the same way before it can be processed. This results in the logic only being executed once on the receive side, instead of once for each target.

- You are using a canonical data model and need a high degree of abstraction from the sending system's format.

- There are many subscribers to a particular message and a high level of abstraction from the sending system is desired.

When a map is bound to a send port, only the target for that specific port will receive the output of the map. No other targets will receive that output unless their send port is configured to call the same map (resulting in the map being called once for each send port bound to it). Bind a map to a send port when:

- Target-specific transformation, translation, or enrichment needs to be performed.

- You are using a canonical data model and need to transform the canonical message to the target-specific format.

Bind a map to an orchestration when:

- Orchestration-specific transformation, translation, or enrichment needs to be performed.

- Multiple maps need to be called in a single subscription.

Binding a Map to a Receive Port

Once your map has been defined, an easy way to execute it is to bind the map to a receive port. To bind a map to a receive port, perform the following steps.

1. Double-click the receive port (not the receive location) in BizTalk Explorer and in the left-hand navigation panel, select **Inbound Maps**.

2. A dialog window appears similar to the one in Figure 4.13. Click on a blank row under the **Map to apply** column. From the combo box, select the map you want to associate to the receive port.

3. Click the **OK** button to close the window.

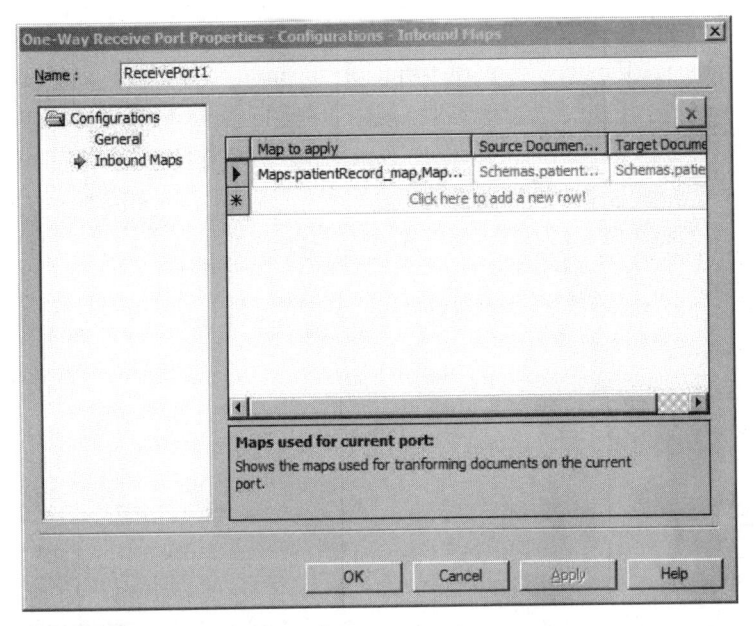

Figure 4.13: Binding a Map to a Receive Port.

> **NOTE**
>
> If you don't see your map in the list, you can apply to a receive port, close the window and refresh the configuration database. Values for BizTalk components available to the server are stored in the configuration database, and sometimes you have to force a refresh for newly-deployed assembly components to be visible. An easy way to refresh the configuration database is to click on the Refresh button at the top of the BizTalk Explorer window.

In Figure 4.13, you'll notice that you can assign multiple maps to a receive port. One common misconception is that this means that the maps are chained. This is not what the receive port configuration dialog box allows you to do. Because a receive port may have multiple receive locations, and thus multiple input formats, you can assign different maps that allow you to map from different input formats to the same output format. This way, if you have a receive port that receives multiple claim formats, they will all be normalized before hitting the message box. If you are in a situation where you need to use multiple maps, you'll need to chain the maps within an orchestration using the Mapping shape.

In order for your map to properly parse the incoming document, you will also need to assign a pipeline to do the message parsing. For information on how to do this, refer to the discussion in Chapter 3 on creating pipelines. Just remember to set the **Document Schema Property** in the flat file disassembler component to the patientRecord.xsd input schema.

Depending on your requirements, maps can also be called from send ports and orchestrations. For more information on orchestrations in BizTalk, see Chapter 5.

Summary

Mapping and metadata are two critical pieces in your BizTalk integration infrastructure. In BizTalk, metadata is defined in XML Schema Definitions, which allow BizTalk to effectively parse and route messages as they flow through the system. Mapping is done in a graphical user interface which leverages the XSLT standard for transformation. These maps allow BizTalk to transform messages so that sending and receiving systems do not have to know what format is required for a particular subscribing system.

Chapter 5

Business Processes & Orchestration

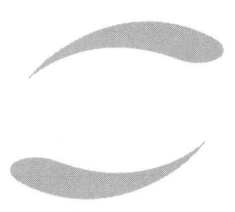

The concept of business activities defined as a set of processes has been around for decades. However, the ability to rapidly define and deploy a business process is a relatively new phenomenon. Totally redesigned in BizTalk 2004, the orchestration functionality is more powerful, scalable, and flexible than ever. Orchestration is a critical part of an enterprise integration architecture that provides a set of graphical tools to define complex interactions, such as correlation across multiple messages, compensating transactions, and rollback.

In this chapter, we will explore what BizTalk orchestration does and how to do some basic configuration with the associated tools.

Web Services—The Building Blocks of Orchestration

Over the past several years, the software industry has been refining an approach to integrating enterprises, applications, and technical components that significantly reduces the cost and complexity of integration. This approach has resulted in the development of a set of standards that build on the lessons learned from previous technology standards such as CORBA, Electronic Data Interchange (EDI), Enterprise Application Integration (EAI), the Internet, and XML. An implementation of this group of standards is collectively referred to as a *web service*. Figure 5.1 shows the anatomy of a web service.

The key advantage to a web service approach over other alternatives such as CORBA is the flexibility and simplicity of the standard itself. For example, the presence of the Internet and ubiquity of HTTP transport allows a web service developer to be freed from the transport or connectivity issues encountered by developers using earlier standards.

Similar to CORBA, a web service is made up of four basic parts:

- **Logic** — Defines the task that the service is supposed to carry out (such as getting status, checking in a patient, and so on), expressed in just about any programming language you choose.

- **Contract** — Expressed in the Web Services Description Language (WSDL), a contract contains the definition of the various methods contained within the service and the inputs/outputs for those methods. WSDLs are defined in XML and are programmatically-accessible documents.

- **Directory/Discovery** — Since services can be located anywhere on a network, a directory service is required for clients to be able to locate the service to be invoked and read the corresponding WSDL. The techniques used to publish the location of a web service, and the protocol through which services are discovered by a client is covered by the Universal Description, Discovery & Integration (UDDI) standard.

- **Transport** — The protocol over which the requests and responses (if any) are exchanged between the web service provider and the web service consumer. Typically, this is the Simple Object Access Protocol (SOAP). Technically speaking, SOAP is really only a lightweight, one-way stateless messaging paradigm, but it is commonly used for request/response scenarios. SOAP is based on XML, is independent of any operating system, and runs on top of any number of lower-level transports, such as HTTP, Java Messaging Service (JMS), or Simple Mail Transport Protocol (SMTP).

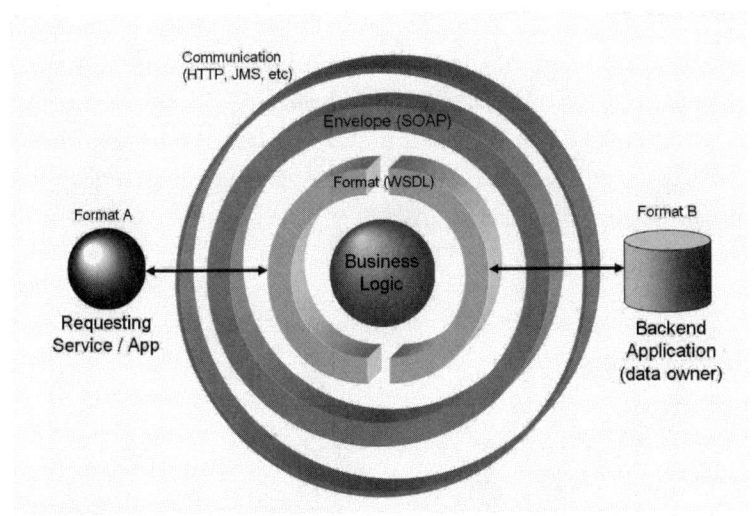

Figure 5.1: Anatomy of a Web Service.

A powerful feature of web services is the ability to aggregate multiple services to create business-level services. For example, if multiple applications need to be updated as the result of a new patient admission into a hospital, each of these individual steps can be rolled into one externally-facing web service method called "admitPatient."

It is this ability to aggregate services that makes web services the "building blocks" for a business-process driven approach to integration projects. But how do you aggregate services? How do you coordinate the complexity associated with correlation, rollback, and timing so you can expose these complex business events as easy-to-use, coarse-grained services? BizTalk orchestration is designed to help us overcome these challenges.

Orchestration—The Foundation for Business Processes

A service-oriented architecture is a loosely-coupled interaction between a requesting entity and one or more responding entities that perform work for the requester. The entities share information about the kind of work they can perform for one another in a programmatically-accessible description language. Orchestration is a vital layer in a service-oriented architecture because it provides the ability to manage complex interactions between multiple services, such as correlation across multiple messages, compensating transactions, and rollback. The functionality provided by orchestration allows for very good abstraction between the technical messaging layer and the business process layer (see Figure 5.2). In very complex integration scenarios, abstraction is a good thing because it results in a more flexible system.

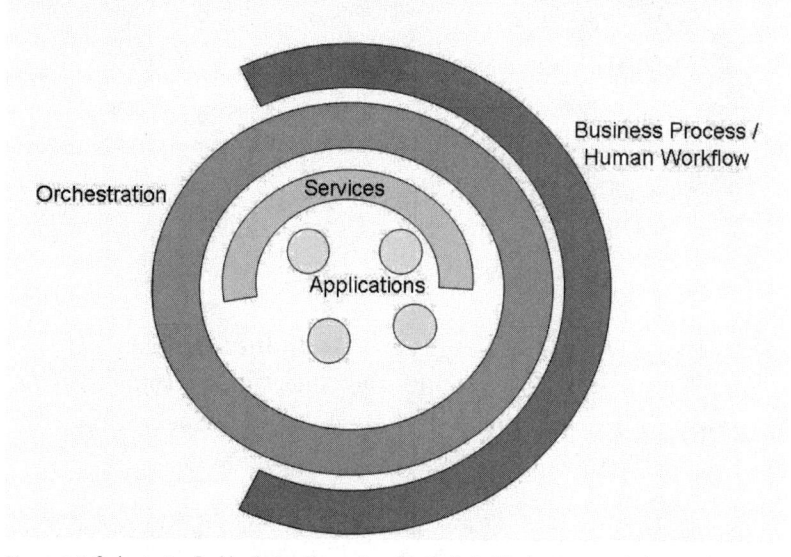

Figure 5.2: Orchestration Enables Proper Abstraction of the Technical Underpinnings of a Service-Oriented Architecture from the Business-Level Process.

> **TIP**
>
> **Because it enables flexibility, proper abstraction is the most important design consideration when building sustainable solutions using service-oriented architectures.**

At its most basic level, orchestration is a state machine shared across multiple services, applications, and/or trading partners. An orchestration schedule defines the flow of events within a business process and keeps track of the state of the message and the participating applications along the way. The end result is a significant reduction in the development effort that was traditionally spent on manually building this functionality into a message broker, database table, or an application. This set of services allows you to build complex business processes that span multiple applications and business partners, without requiring significant programming skills.

Orchestrations are defined in a proprietary XML format called XLANG/S, but can be imported or exported via the industry-standard Business Process Execution Language (BPEL) for use in any BPEL-compliant design tool. BizTalk Server provides a graphical user interface called the Orchestration Designer, which is hosted within the Visual Studio .NET integrated design environment (IDE).

> **⚠ CAUTION**
>
> **Special care has to be taken when creating a BPEL-compliant process, because BizTalk orchestration provides many more features and capabilities than the current standard for BPEL can describe.**

A common goal of many integration projects is the definition of an end-to-end process for a major area of the business. For example, setting up a new group at an insurance provider involves multiple people, systems, and departments. Once defined, an enterprise business process can give business users total visibility into the business and dramatically increase the agility of how that process is carried out. Unfortunately, actually implementing an enterprise business process is usually just as futile as a search for the Holy Grail. The problem is a lack of abstraction. While it is a straightforward discussion to define an enterprise business process, there are too many moving parts to be coordinated and too many interfaces and messages to be managed by a single project.

However, with an orchestration layer, the multitude of touch points and other complexities can be greatly reduced for the business process. Instead of managing 50 applications and 100 interfaces, a business process can interact with just a couple of orchestrations. This is a much more realistic proposition, and will greatly increase your chances of success for this type of project.

Incidentally, the business process layer itself could be composed of a macro-orchestration, a human workflow services schedule, or a Microsoft partner's business process product such as Metastorm's e-Work.

When to Use Orchestration

BizTalk orchestration provides the services that enable you to design, deploy, and manage business processes. While it is not a required component for all of your integration scenarios, an orchestration is a powerful piece of the BizTalk Server stack that is best used under the following conditions:

- **Long running processes** — When a process takes hours, days, or even weeks to complete, correlating events can become very difficult. When dealing with a long running process, it can be a challenge for a developer to properly write code that would manage the resources and state for that process. Through processes known as dehydration and rehydration, processes and state are persisted to a database until the time comes where they can continue processing. By leveraging this feature, orchestrations can be used to automatically handle this task for you. For example, if you send more than 1000 messages via the Internet, you would not want 1000 running threads waiting indefinitely for a response.

- **Complex flow logic** — If your process can fork into multiple paths, it may be beneficial to use an orchestration to define when and how the process might go down one path versus another.

- **Integration with other BizTalk modules without code** — Through an orchestration, you can more easily use a number of other Microsoft services without the need to write code. If you are looking for an easily maintained method for incorporating the following services, an orchestration is the way to go.

    o *Web Services* — SOAP-based connectivity for bi-directional communication with web services can be automatically generated by drag and drop configuration and basic property configuration in the Orchestration Designer.

    o *Business Activity Monitoring (BAM)* — A set of tools for information workers to monitor transactions and processes in real time. Chapter 6 covers BAM in detail.

    o *Business Rules Framework* — Core functionality for defining, managing, and deploying complex business rules used for one or many business processes across the organization.

How to Use and Configure Orchestrations in BizTalk

This section explores the basics of orchestrations in BizTalk 2004. A number of significant improvements have been included in the 2004 release, making orchestrations scalable, robust, and more powerful. Since orchestration and business process management is such a broad topic, the next few pages are intended to give you a feel for the major pieces and concepts behind orchestration.

Creating Orchestrations

Rebuilt in BizTalk Server 2004, the Orchestration Designer is now integrated into Visual Studio .NET. To start working with a new orchestration, right click on a new or existing BizTalk project in the Solution Explorer and select **Add New Item**. As shown in Figure 5.3, click on an orchestration and give it a name. Click the **Open** button.

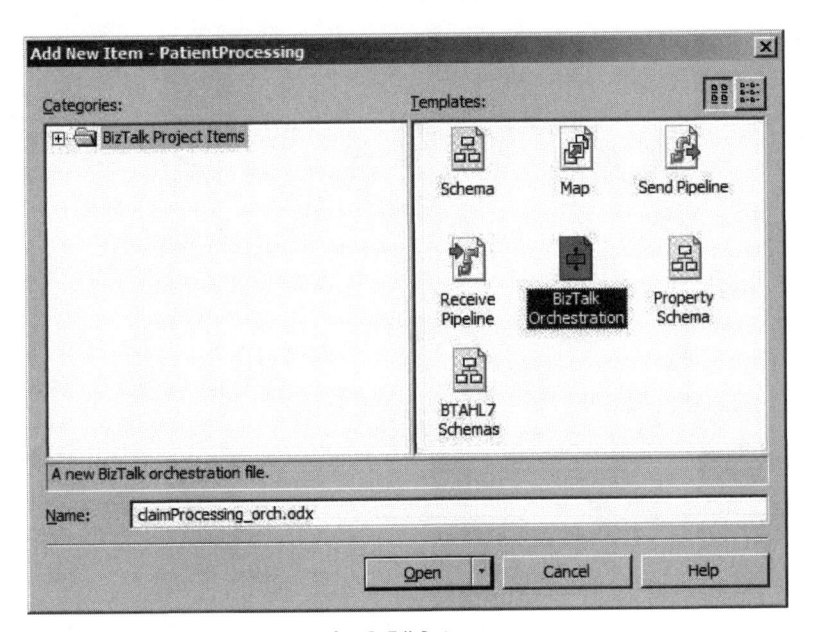

Figure 5.3: Creating a New Orchestration for a BizTalk Project.

> **TIP**
>
> A good way to organize your integration scenario is to separate it into projects based on the type of component. For example, create a project that just contains orchestrations. Remember to add in the necessary references to required assemblies such as schemas and maps if you use this approach.

After you have added the new orchestration, the Orchestration Designer will appear in Visual Studio .NET, as shown in Figure 5.4.

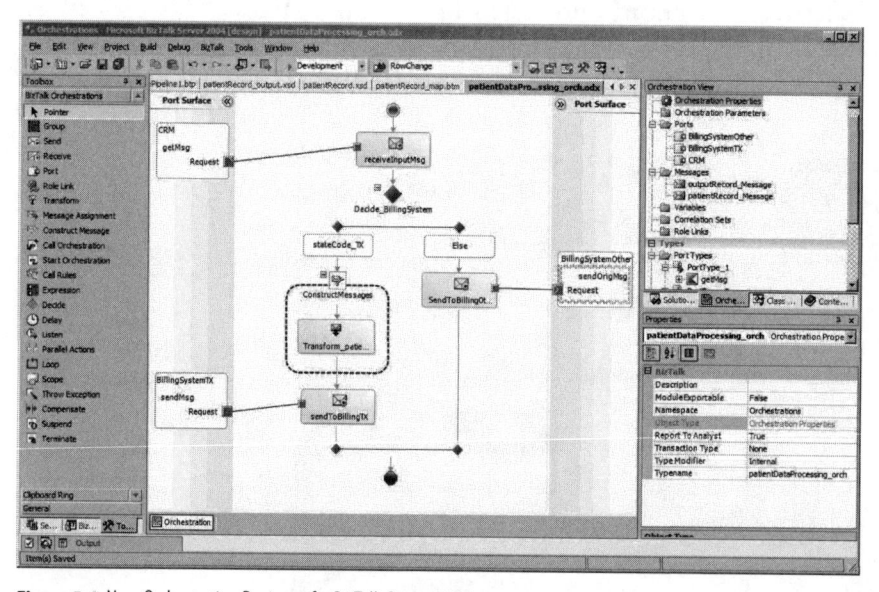

Figure 5.4: New Orchestration Designer for BizTalk Server 2004.

The Orchestration Designer is composed of four types of windows.

- **Orchestration Toolbox** — Holds the shapes which can be placed into the other windows to graphically define your business process. Drag and drop shapes from the toolbox onto either the orchestration workspace or port surfaces to build your business process. The Orchestration Toolbox is shown in Figure 5.5.

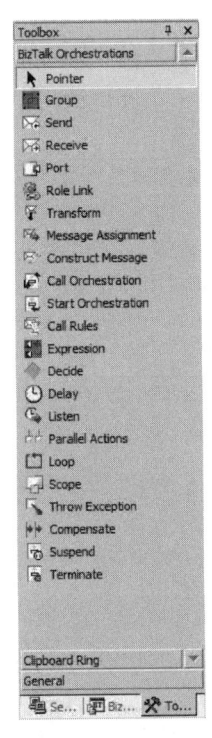

Figure 5.5: Orchestration Toolbox.

- **Orchestration workspace** — This is the centermost part of the screen. It contains the definition of business and integration logic that defines your process, as shown in Figure 5.6.

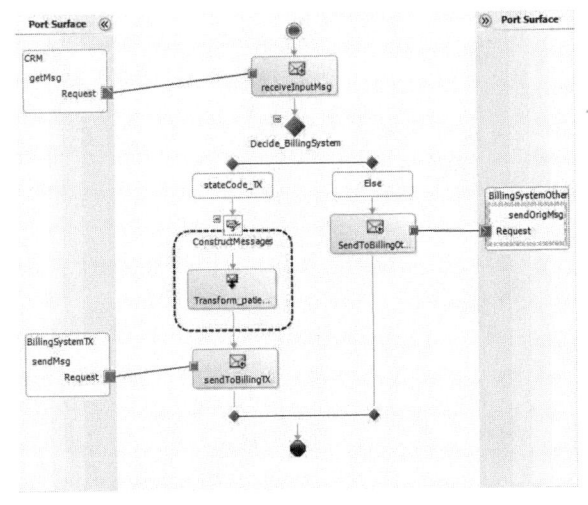

Figure 5.6: Orchestration Workspace.

The workspace is composed of a center area where the process flow is defined, plus two port surfaces on either side. These areas hold the logical port definitions that will connect the orchestration to physical endpoints. It does not matter which port surface window you choose to place your ports.

- **Orchestration View** — Contains all of the objects that the orchestration uses to connect to ports and process messages, as shown in Figure 5.7. The most common objects include:

  o **Messages** — These represent an individual instance of a message defined by a schema. All messages must be defined in this way to the orchestration and bound to a schema in order to be processed by the orchestration.

  o **Ports** — These are abstract representations of a physical send or receive port. If you select **Specify Later** for the port binding during the creation of the port, you are not required to define a physical port until the orchestration is enlisted by the server.

  o **Variables** — These hold values that are defined and used by the business process itself.

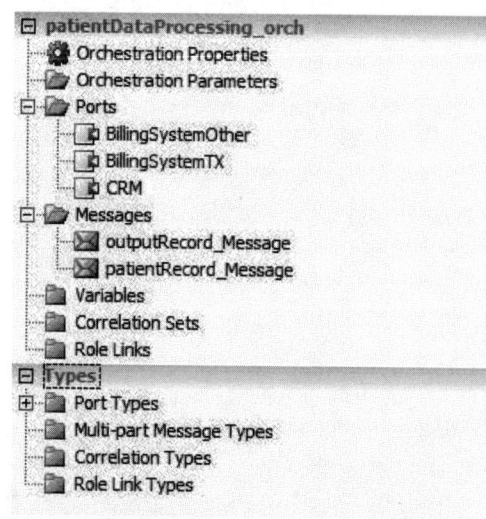

Figure 5.7: Orchestration View.

- **Properties Window** — As shown in Figure 5.8, this window holds the configuration information for shapes placed on the orchestration workspace, as well as objects defined in the Orchestration View. If you're familiar with Visual Studio, this window is nothing new.

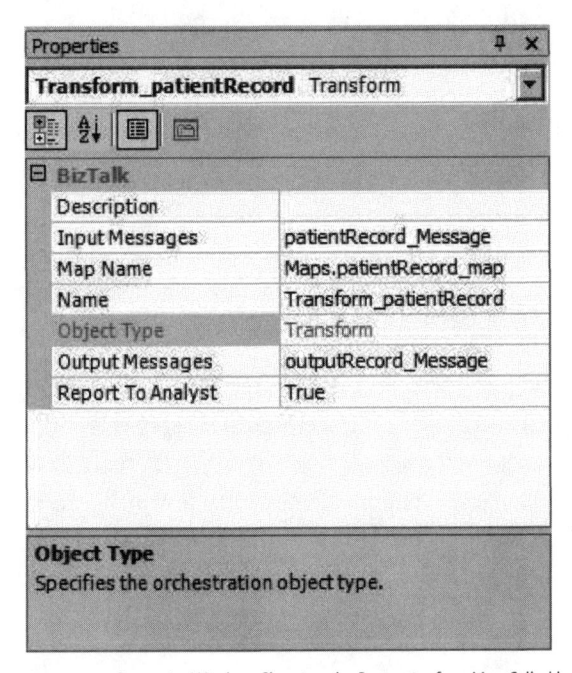

Figure 5.8: Properties Window, Showing the Properties for a Map Called by an Orchestration.

Configuring Orchestrations for Runtime

Once the process flow has been defined in the Orchestration Designer, the schedule is ready to be deployed. The process of deployment for an orchestration schedule is the same as for other BizTalk artifacts. From the **Tools** menu in Visual Studio .NET, select **Deploy**. Once deployed, you must bind any logical send and receive ports used in the orchestration to actual send and receive ports on the server. This is done by right-clicking on the orchestration in BizTalk Explorer and selecting **Bind**.

Once all ports have been bound in the orchestration, it is ready to start. In BizTalk Explorer, you can start an orchestration by right-clicking on the orchestration and selecting **Start**. The icon will change from black and white to a colored icon once the schedule has been started successfully.

Advanced Orchestration Concepts

The BizTalk community is constantly discovering new ways to utilize orchestrations for complex integration scenarios and business processes. An excellent resource for the latest information and techniques on orchestration is a blog by Scott Woodgate, Lead Product Manager for BizTalk Server. You can access his blog through http://blogs.msdn.com.

Here, we will discuss some of the more common concepts that can greatly enhance the way in which you use orchestration in your projects.

Correlation

You will often have messages in a business process that are related based on the content of the messages themselves. *Correlation* is the relationship between individual messages based on content. Defining relationships between separate messages is handled by *correlation sets*. To build a correlation between messages, you must first create a correlation type by right-clicking on correlation types in the orchestration view and selecting **New Correlation Type**. The **Correlation Properties** window appears, as shown in Figure 5.9.

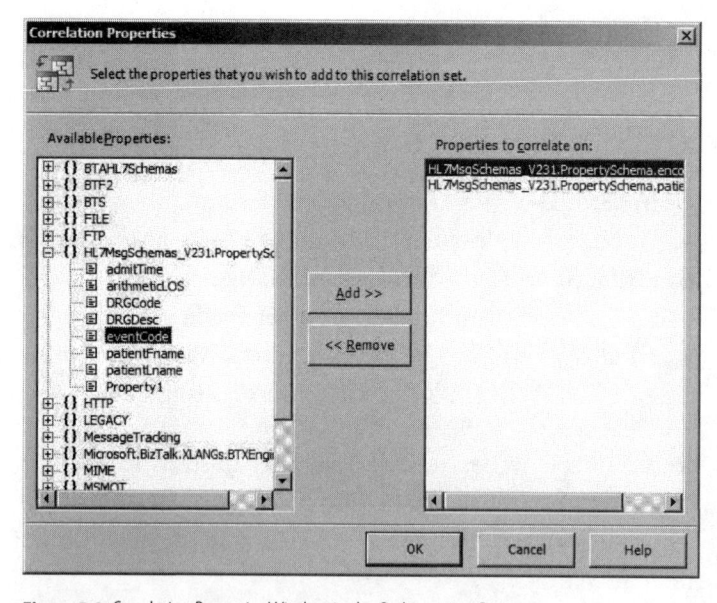

Figure 5.9: Correlation Properties Window in the Orchestration Designer.

The available fields on which to create the correlation are system variables, BizTalk standard variables, and promoted properties. The most common correlations are based on a promoted property. Promoting a property creates a copy of the data held in that element in a globally accessible part of the message box. By using promoted properties, the format and type of the message is abstracted, and only the value of that field is used to build the correlation. For more information on how to promote a property in a message schema, see Chapter 4.

Once the correlation type has been created, the next step is to create an instance of that type in the schedule. This instance is called a correlation set, and is created by right-clicking on the **Correlation Set** folder icon in the Orchestration View. Select **New Correlation Set** and select the appropriate correlation type.

We have now bound a promoted property to a correlation type and then bound that type to the schedule through the creation of a correlation set. The next step is to bind the correlation set to all of the Receive shapes that handle the inbound messages that make up the convoy. This is done by setting the **Initializing Correlation Set** property in the Receive shape to the appropriate value.

It is important to note that by creating a correlation between messages, no modifications are made to the message content itself. The use of correlation is completely transparent to systems outside of BizTalk.

Transaction and Compensation

Orchestrations and orchestration components can either be *long-running* or *atomic* transactions.

Atomic — The entire orchestration is rolled back if any step fails.

Long running — If a step fails, rollback is not performed, but compensating transactions can be implemented.

To set an entire orchestration schedule to be long-running or atomic, set the **Transaction Type** property, as shown in Figure 5.10

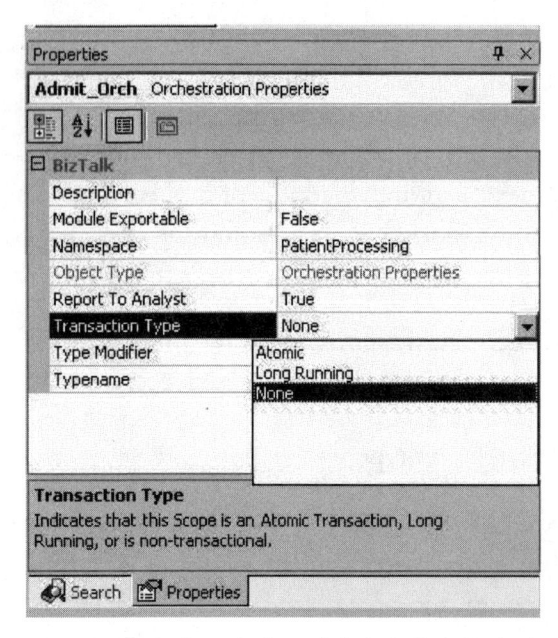

Figure 5.10: Setting Transaction Type in Orchestration Properties.

Convoy

A *convoy* is a type of correlation that is a group of related messages identified by a field or group of fields within each message. The first message in the convoy defines the values that will be used to define whether or not subsequent messages are included in the set. For example, all messages that contain the same social security number are related in a particular encounter process, regardless of the format of the message.

A convoy of messages must also be processed by the same instance in order to be valid. For example, if a patient admission for someone with an SSN of 123-45-6789 starts an orchestration schedule, only a discharge for a patient with an SSN of 123-45-6789 will be consumed.

There are three basic types of convoys: Parallel, Uniform Sequential, and Non-Uniform Sequential. Let's take a closer look at each.

Parallel Convoy

In a parallel convoy, a set of related messages may arrive in any order. However, all messages must be received in order for the process to be valid. The messages can be of different types, and the arrival of any type of message will trigger the process.

To implement a parallel convoy, drag a Parallel Action shape onto the palette, with a fork for each of the messages that make up the convoy. Define a correlation set and bind it to each Receive shape. Figure 5.11 shows two messages in a convoy.

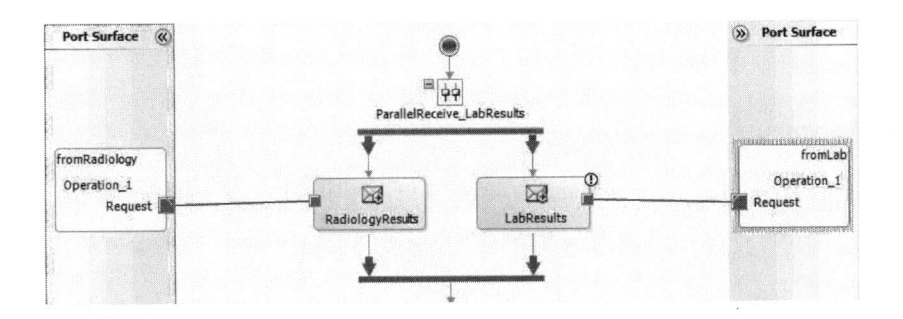

Figure 5.11: A Parallel Convoy.

Uniform Sequential Convoy

In a uniform sequential convoy, a set of the same message type is received from the same source. No predefined order exists, so the messages should be processed sequentially as they arrive.

This technique makes use of the Loop shape. Since all messages are of the same type, the same Receive shape can be used inside of the loop. If, for instance, we expect four messages to make up the set, the loop can be hard-coded to complete after four messages are received. If there is a value that is calculated or derived from data in the message, the loop argument can be set to that expression. Be sure to set the Receive shape's **Initializing Correlation** property appropriately. A uniform sequential convoy is shown in Figure 5.12.

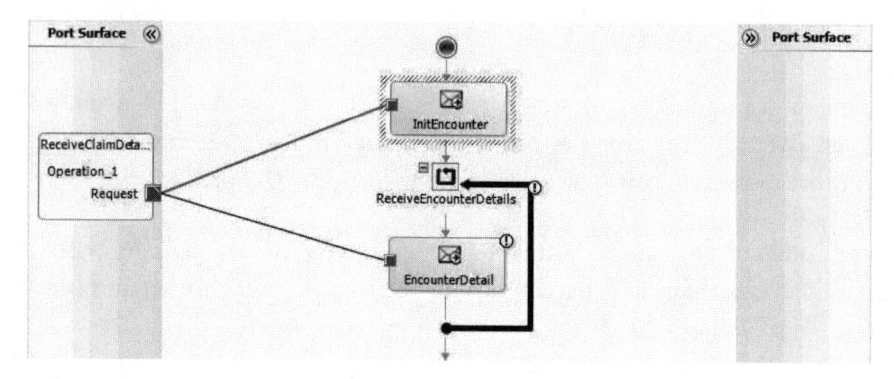

Figure 5.12: A Uniform Sequential Convoy.

Non-Uniform Sequential Convoy

In a non-uniform sequential convoy, messages of different types arrive in a predetermined order. If messages are received out of order, an error is thrown.

This technique makes use of the multiple operation feature of receive ports. To add an operation to a receive port, right-click on the shape and select **Add Operation**. Follow the prompts in the wizard. Next, create a Receive shape for each message that will arrive and be sure to place them in the order in which they are expected to arrive. Set the **Initializing Correlation** property for the first Receive shape appropriately. A non-uniform sequential convoy is shown in Figure 5.13.

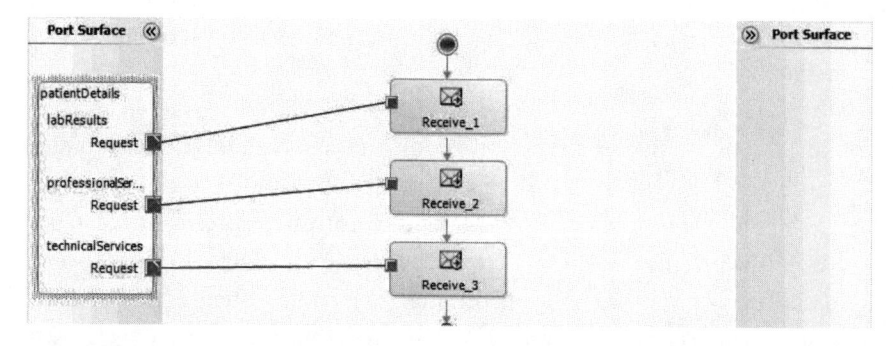

Figure 5.13: A Non-Uniform Sequential Convoy.

Summary

Perhaps the biggest change between the BizTalk Server 2004 release and previous releases is the new set of capabilities in the orchestration layer. Orchestration is a key enabler for enterprise business processes and service-oriented architectures. It defines coarse-grained business events and processes ranging from the basic to the highly complex. Architects should think twice before dismissing this layer as "fluff." They should consider orchestration to be the lynchpin between the plumbing of the EAI world and the high-level services of human workflow, business process management, and business activity monitoring.

Did you know?

You can automatically deploy orchestrations, port configurations, and other components from the command line or programmatically.

A set of utilities installed in <BizTalk home directory>\SDK\WMI can be used as part of a batch script to allow for error-free migration to other BizTalk server environments. All you need is a binding file for your orchestration and the assembly that contains the orchestration. The binding file contains configuration information required by the server for deployment and can be created by executing the BizTalk Deployment wizard, which is located from in the BizTalk Server 2004 program group in the Start menu.

Each of the SDK utilities comes with well-commented code, so it's easy for you to modify to fit your needs.

You can also use a file called Setup.bat (in the SDK directory) to automatically deploy and start your orchestrations.

Chapter 6

Business Activity Monitoring

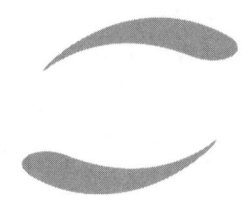

A recent survey of business executives found that the majority felt that IT has become an inhibitor to growth. In fact, 203 of the 359 participants said that lack of information was a key reason that IT was holding back growth.

Part of the problem is that business people need a different view into the business than technically-oriented monitoring tools can provide. Traditionally, batch-driven reports are the only means for knowledge workers to gain a business-oriented view into their processes. But in today's fast-paced business climate, an event-driven, near real-time insight into the business is required. After all, knowledge workers need information they can use to better the business, not documentation of where processes went wrong last quarter.

Business activity monitoring (BAM) is the culmination of several years of effort by the software industry to provide businesses with a near real-time view into key performance criteria, regardless of which application or applications are handling the activity. Technically speaking, BAM is about intercepting, aggregating and analyzing technical events along with business data in near real-time to provide a business-oriented view into your processes.

What is a Business Activity?

At the heart of business activity monitoring (BAM) is the concept of, you guessed it, a business activity. Unlike technically-oriented events, such as raising an error condition, or the appearance of a message in a queue, a business activity is the intersection of data, business and process logic, and context. A graphical depiction of the relationship between these elements in a business activity is shown in Figure 6.1.

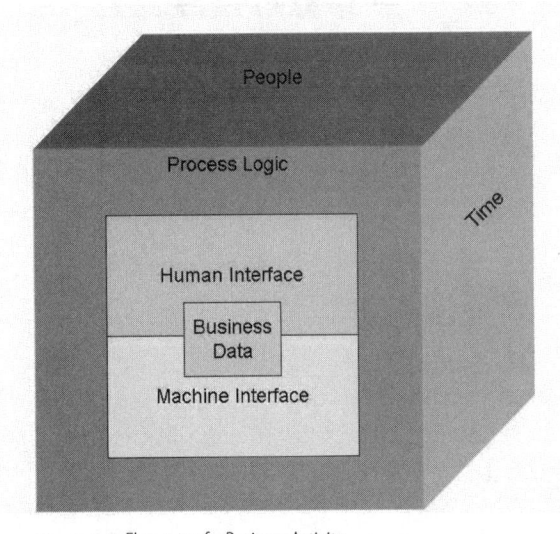

Figure 6.1: Elements of a Business Activity.

Since most systems are not designed with this kind of underlying concept, it can be very difficult to accurately translate technical events and data into meaningful, business-level activities. In addition, the data and technical events that make up business activities will often span multiple applications, making it even more difficult to build a business activity from existing systems.

BAM and Business Process Integration

As a result of these challenges, BAM has been a pipe dream until the arrival of an affordable, easily maintained business process integration platform, such as BizTalk Server 2004 combined with the powerful analytics (OLAP) capabilities of SQL Server 2000. With a business process integration platform in place, we can handle and recognize technical events regardless of whether or not they occur in one application or many. Using orchestration, we can aggregate these technical events along with the corresponding data to build the foundation that will allow the definition of business activities.

A Framework for BAM

So how can you take business data, process-oriented data, and combine them in a way that results in the creation of a business activity? A first step is to look at BAM as a layered technology, as depicted in Figure 6.2.

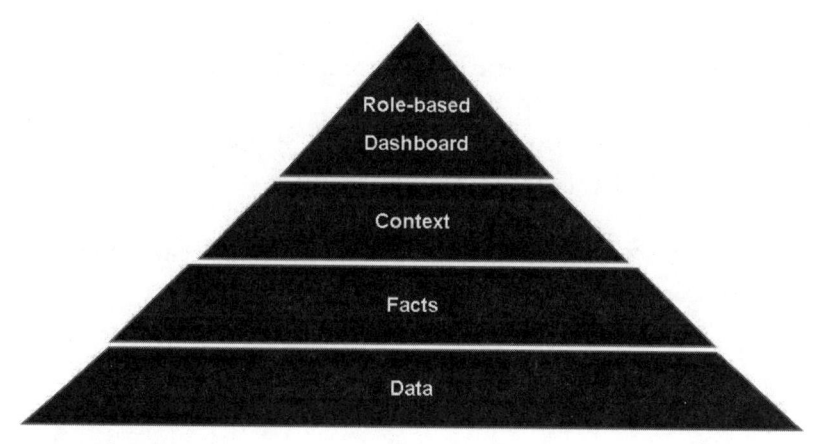

Figure 6.2: The BAM Pyramid.

Let's examine each layer.

Data

The foundation of the pyramid is data. In this case, data refers to the hundreds of thousands of bits of information scattered throughout an enterprise. An example of raw data might be a patient name or a claim number.

Facts

Facts are groupings of related data that allow us to make statements about the business. An example of a fact would be that lab technician John Doe purchased $100,000 worth of medical supplies from the company.

Context

Context refers to the circumstances within which an event occurs. Facts are closely related to context. Facts can be an event or transaction, while the context is the setting in which that transaction or event took place.

Expanding on our previous example, we can take related pieces of data (a lab technician and a purchase order of lab equipment), put them together to create a fact (John Doe bought $50 of lab equipment), and then collect information about when, how, and why this fact occurred to get context. For example, John Doe bought $50 of equipment last Tuesday from our Internet site because there was an increase in the number of patients that had a certain medical condition.

Facts are often given with no context, which can result in misleading and inaccurate information. Consider the following fact: in 1973, baseball hall-of-fame pitcher Nolan Ryan set the record for the most strikeouts in a single season (383), had a very respectable earned run average of 2.87, and had a record of 21 wins and 16 losses.

But when you take into account the rest of the team's performance, you can understand that in fact the 1973 Angels had a losing season that year.

The goal of context is to give meaning to facts, so that business people can make informed decisions based on reality, and not a mish-mash of data.

Dashboard

Once you have the context for a set of facts, that information should be accessible to a business user in an easily understood way. This is often accomplished using charts, spreadsheets, or other techniques to communicate information in a familiar and easily displayed environment.

Dashboards are the user interface layer and represent the final component to the BAM framework. Much like the dashboard on your car, the idea here is to boil a lot of information down to an easily understood set of "gauges" that give the user real-time information about the overall health of the business, department, or team.

Business Activity Monitoring with BizTalk Server 2004

This section will focus on two approaches to implementing BAM with BizTalk Server 2004. Information resources that deal with the nuts and bolts behind Microsoft's BAM implementation can be found in the "Further Resources" section at the end of the book. The purpose of this section will be to introduce you to the technology and illustrate the linkages specific to BizTalk.

When to Use Business Activity Monitoring with BizTalk

BAM is intended to be used by information workers within the enterprise who need a real-time view into their business processes. Utilizing BAM assumes that there is an active business process, (or orchestration in BizTalk terms) running within the organization. (For more information on building an orchestration, see Chapter 5). Information workers need not necessarily be IT professionals, nor should it be assumed that they are technologically proficient. As a result, this technology is a good fit when:

- You have a business user who expresses the need to know what's going on in his or her department.

- The business user is using BizTalk Server to route and integrate messages and processes.

- The business user is comfortable using Excel pivot tables.

Building the BAM Definition

Once you have identified the need and fit for a BAM solution, the first step is to determine what data, facts, and context need to be represented in the dashboard.

To properly define these criteria, a BAM definition file must be created. These files are built using an Excel spreadsheet template included with the installation of the Business Activity Monitoring infrastructure. This spreadsheet contains several macros that provide the links to the BAM server. In a default installation, this spreadsheet is called BAM.xls.

Typically, a knowledge worker will make a copy of this spreadsheet, and build a "wish list" of data and facts to build a report on. The knowledge worker will do this by walking through a wizard-driven interface accessible within the spreadsheet. The next few sections will walk you through how to define the "wish list." At a high level, the knowledge worker will define the key activities to be monitored at an abstract level, and then define how to structure the information in a view.

The nice thing about this approach is that business users can define their needs using the familiar user experience of Excel. The resulting definition is at an abstract level, so the knowledge worker does not need to know how or where that data is coming from.

> **TIP**
>
> While a file can hold multiple activities, only one view can be stored in each spreadsheet, so you should name the spreadsheet files after a view.

Building a Business Activity

The first step is to define the business activities that form the foundation for our view. A *business activity* is a collection of related data, facts, and context all rolled into one.

Use the following procedure to define a business activity.

1. Open the BAM.xls spreadsheet. From the **BAM** menu, choose **BAM Activity**, as shown in Figure 6.3.

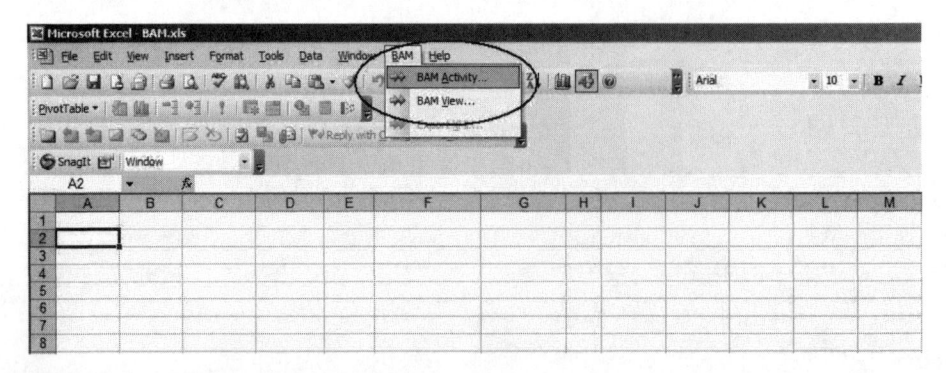

Figure 6.3: Select BAM Activity from the BAM Menu.

2. The **BAM Activity** wizard will open. Click the button labeled **New Activity** and you will see a screen similar to Figure 6.4. Type in the name of your activity. In this case, let's build an activity that will define the data and context associated with admitting a new patient.

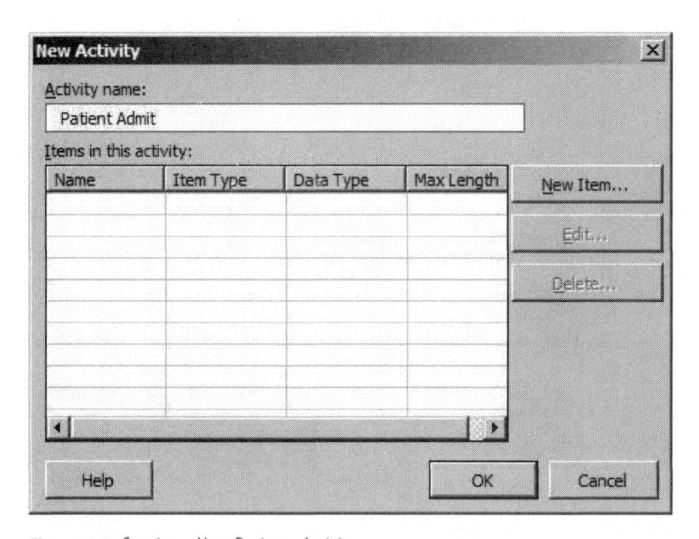

Figure 6.4: Creating a New Business Activity.

3. To build a set of related data around the activity, click the **New Item** button. Give the item a name and then you can select one of several item types (see Figure 6.5).

   - **Business Milestone** — Defines a time context associated with the activity, such as the beginning or ending time of an event.

   - **Business Data – Text** — Assigned to text elements that should be displayed in the view.

   - **Business Data – Integer** — Assigned to calculated and/or displayed integer elements that should be displayed in the view.

   - **Business Data – Float** — Same as integer elements but used with float data types.

   Keep in mind that items are not limited to only the data that appears on a single message or even any message at all. At this point, all that's being done is defining what data and context needs to be part of the view.

Computations such as average, minimum, maximum, and so on can all be done within the BAM infrastructure. BAM can also correlate multiple messages, processes, and data sources (using BizTalk), so do not feel that your view is limited to the data that exists in a particular message.

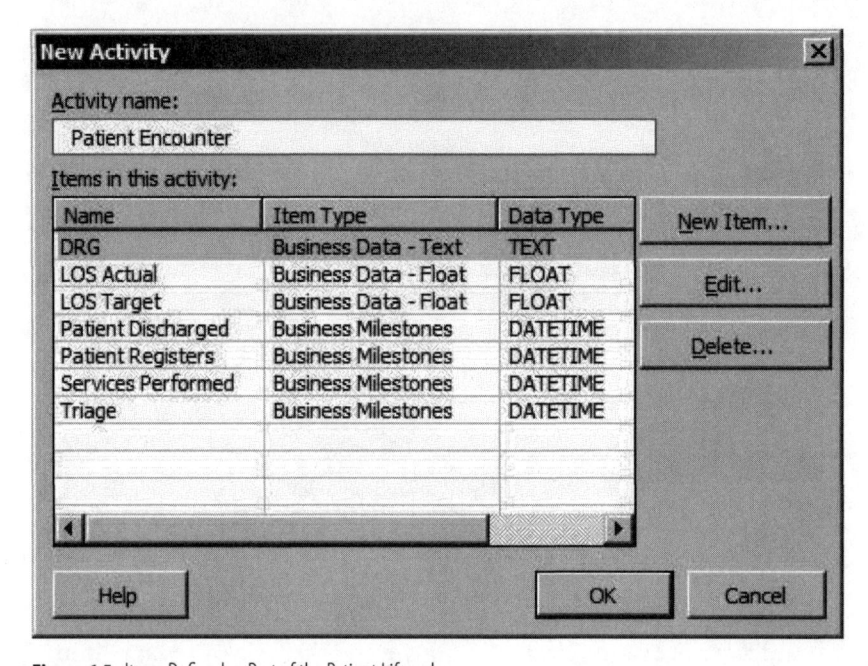

Figure 6.5: Items Defined as Part of the Patient Lifecycle.

4. Once you have finished entering all of the aspects of the activity, click the **OK** button. If you have other activities that make up the view you anticipate building, you can define them. Otherwise, click the **OK** button again to complete building business activities.

Building a Business Activity Monitoring View

Once you have defined the business activity or activities you want to monitor, you need to define how you want information about the activity presented. Use the following procedure to build a BAM view.

1. Select **BAM View** from the **BAM** menu, or, if you just created a BAM activity, you will automatically be taken to the **BAM View** wizard shown in Figure 6.6.

Chapter 6 - Business Activity Monitoring

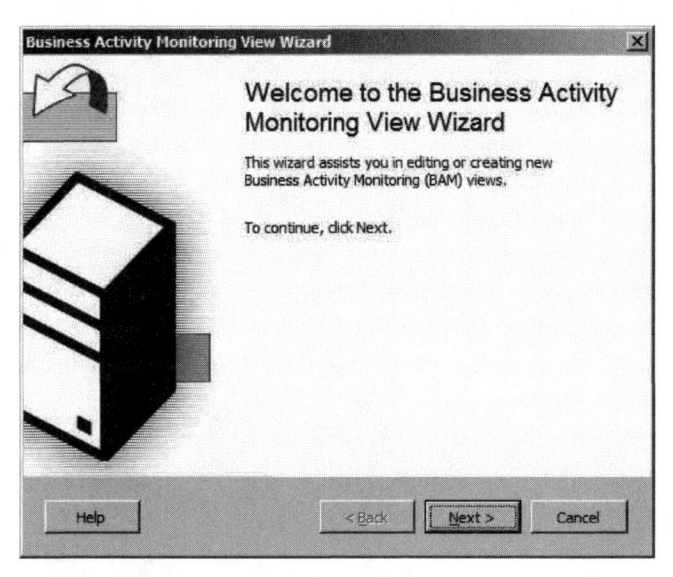

Figure 6.6: BAM View Wizard.

2. Click the **Next** button, and a screen appears where you can create, edit, or delete views that are associated with the current workbook.

> **TIP**
>
> **If you need to delete a view that you have already deployed to the server, make sure to delete the view from the server as well using the bm.exe command-line tool (covered later this chapter).**

3. Click the **Next** button again to create a new view and give it a logical name. As shown in Figure 6.7, select the activities to be included in the view and click the **Next** button.

105

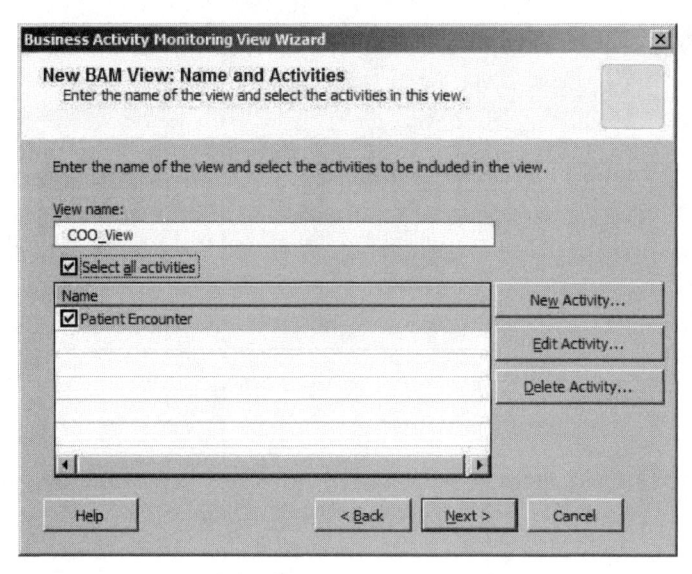

Figure 6.7: Activities to Include in BAM View.

4. The next step in the wizard will prompt you to select the items from the activities you chose previously. Depending on how you have structured your view(s), you may not want to have all items included (see Figure 6.8).

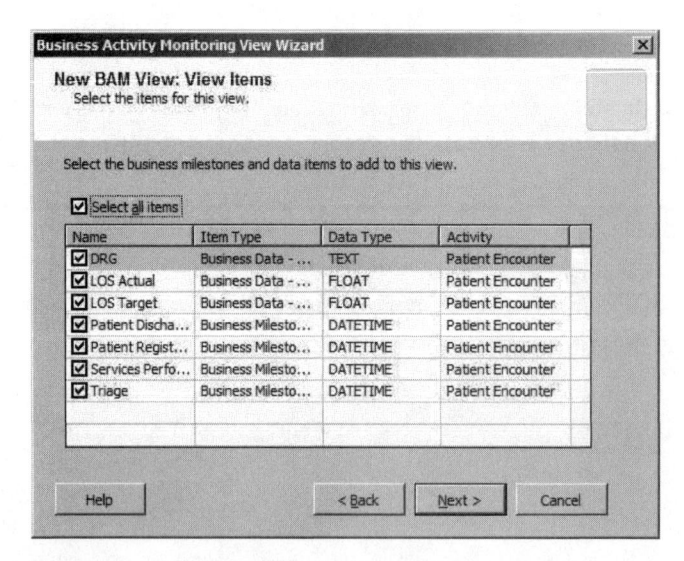

Figure 6.8: Items to Include in the View.

5. The next step is very important to building your view. This is where you build facts and context from the individual data points. Here, you will build relationships between, for example, the admit time and the discharge time to define the length of stay. Figure 6.9 shows a duration being defined for the length-of-stay for a patient visit.

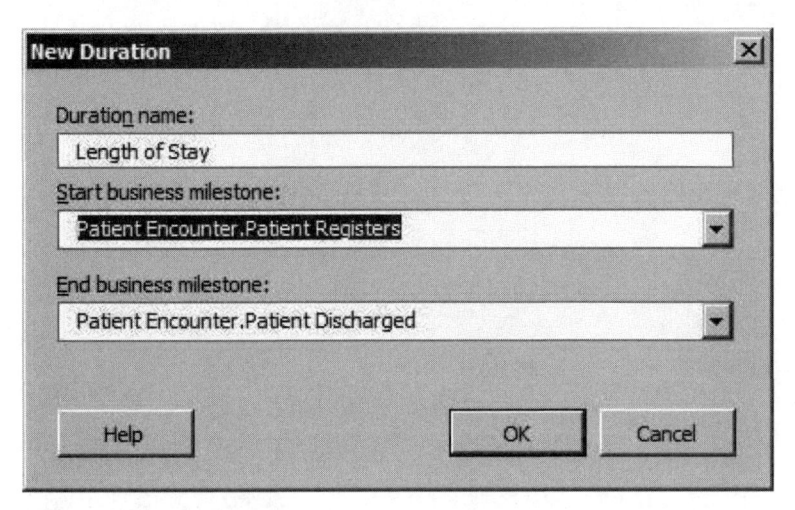

Figure 6.9: Defining a New Duration.

6. Once you have built all of the relationships between the data, click the **Next** button. The next screen displayed in the **BAM View** wizard allows you to define aggregation dimensions and measures. Aggregating information is a key to building the dashboard layer of the BAM framework. Here, you can take large amounts of complex data and start to make it more easily managed from a high level to get an overall view of the business.

There are two ways to aggregate information in BAM: *dimensions* and *measures*. By clicking on the button labeled **New Dimension**, or the one labeled **New Measure**, the wizard will walk you through the process of how the information will be aggregated and displayed to the end user. Let's take a closer look at how to use dimensions and measures.

- **New Dimension**

    o **Progress** — As shown in Figure 6.10, a progress dimension is used to describe the lifecycle of a business process, such as the stage of a patient in an encounter (triage, awaiting surgery, discharge, etc.).

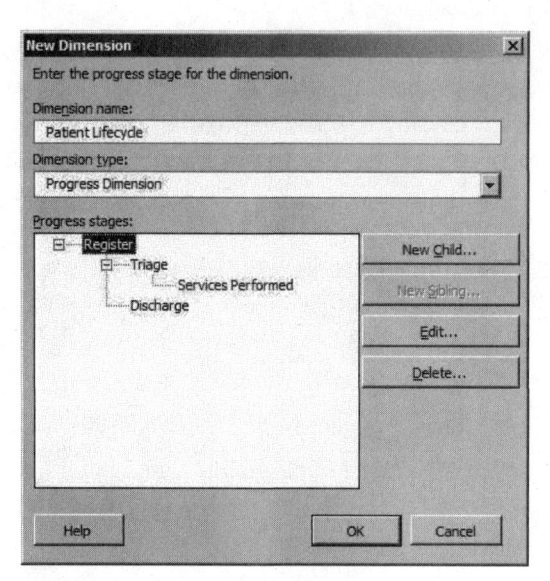

Figure 6.10: Defining a new Dimension.

- o   **Data** — Allows the view to be built around a particular data element, such as a listing by Diagnosis Related Group (DRG) code.

- o   **Numeric Range Dimension** — Defines ranges to be assigned, typically in low/medium/high groupings. For example, claims below $1000 are grouped as low, while claims of $1000 and above are high.

- o   **Time Dimension** — Used to display information sorted by base business milestones.

- **New Measure** — Allows you to perform aggregate functions on items and sets of related items (such as duration). For example, a measure allows you to calculate the average length of stay across all patient encounters, or a subset of encounters, such as diagnosis code. Figure 6.11 shows a measure of average length of stay being defined.

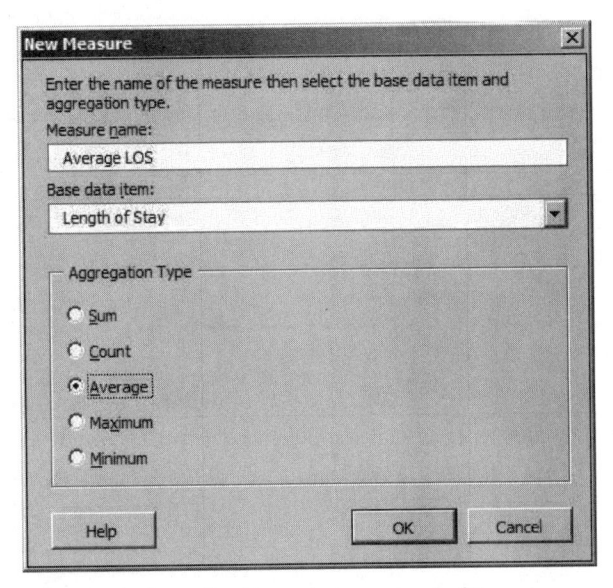

Figure 6.11: Defining a New Measure for Average Length of Stay.

7. Once you have defined all of your measures and aggregation dimensions, click the **Next** button and a confirmation screen will be displayed by the wizard, as shown in Figure 6.12.

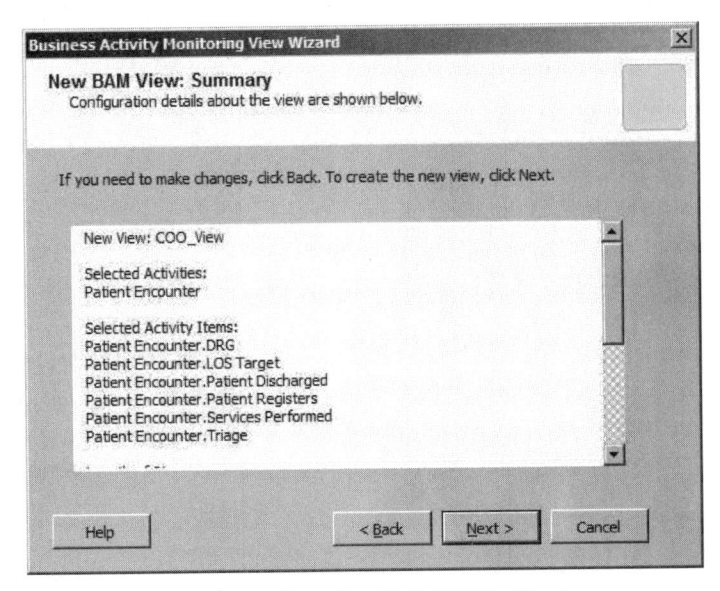

Figure 6.12: Confirming Items and View Created in the BAM View Wizard.

8. Click the **Next** button to exit the wizard. Once the wizard closes, a familiar pivot table layout will appear in the Excel worksheet. Now you can drag and drop items onto the pivot table to build the initial report structure that will be displayed to the user. At this point, your BAM definition file is ready to be deployed to the BAM infrastructure.

> **NOTE**
>
> You will notice that information is populated into the table as soon as you drop elements into it. This data is just mocked-up for you to get a feel for what the report will look like once deployed. It is not actual data from your process.

Deploying a BAM Definition File

Technically speaking, a BAM definition holds the schema for the database objects that are created to store the context and business data that you want to track.

Before you deploy the BAM definition file you defined in the previous section to the server, you need to make a decision. Do you want to have the information available in real-time or can you afford to wait a little bit and have the ability to slice and dice the information in more ways?

You can choose from the following options.

Deployment Option 1: Real-Time Aggregation (RTA)

If you choose to monitor in real-time, the BAM infrastructure will create a set of relational tables in SQL Server. To enable RTA, click on an area on the pivot table, and click the **RTA** button that is part of the pivot table toolbar, as shown in Figure 6.13. You will know that RTA is enabled when the button has a thin black outline around it.

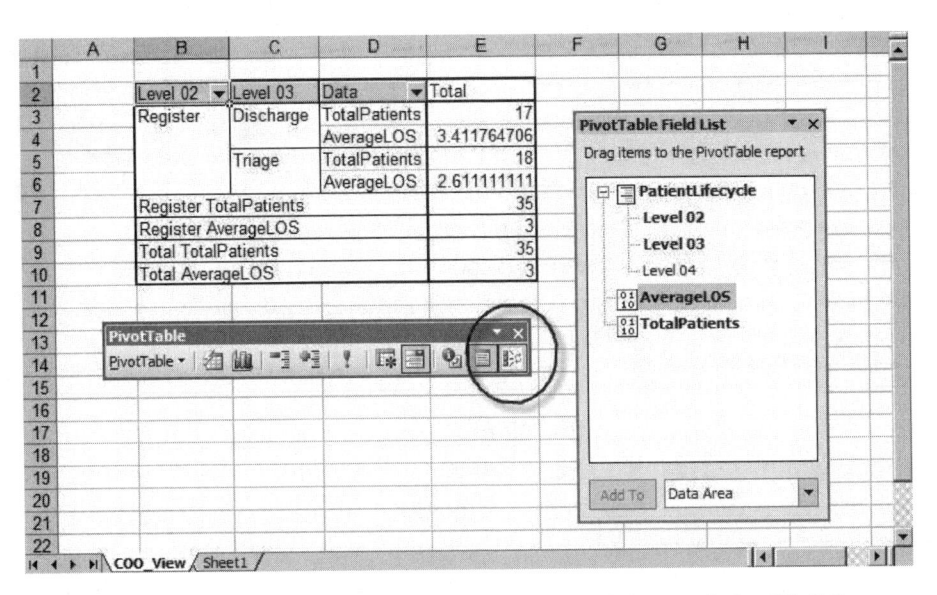

Figure 6.13: Selecting a BAM View for Real-Time Aggregation by Clicking the RTA Button on the Pivot Table Toolbar.

Deployment Option 2: OLAP Cube

On the other hand, if you want more flexibility and power in the reporting options, you can have the BAM infrastructure create an Online Analytical Processing (OLAP) cube to store the information as part of SQL Server Analysis Services. This option also allows you to manage limited network and hardware resources in situations with high message volume by batching updates to the BAM tables. If you choose this option, you will need to process the cube before the pivot table will be populated in Excel. A best practice for this approach is to schedule a job in SQL to automatically process the cube on a regular basis. Since this is the default option, all you need to do is make sure that the **RTA** button on the pivot table toolbar is not selected. You will know that RTA is not enabled when the button has no thin black outline around it.

> **TIP**
>
> A real-time aggregation may degrade performance in some integration scenarios because the system will be actively updating the BAM tables in real-time. In situations where many messages are flowing through the system and RTA is required, plan on adding hardware resources (such as memory, CPUs, servers, faster disk) to compensate. Only choose real-time if required by the business or if the anticipated load is low enough that the impact will not matter.

Usually, an information worker can handle all of the previous steps without too much difficulty, and the completed Excel spreadsheet is given to the BizTalk developer. It is at this stage that the actual data elements are mapped into the view and the BAM definition is deployed to the server.

Using the BAM Deployment Tool

From a command prompt, navigate to the directory <BizTalk Installation Dir>\Tracking. This directory holds a number of configuration files and other objects that make up most of the BAM infrastructure. To deploy our BAM definition, you need to use the BAM deployment tool (bm.exe).

> **TIP**
>
> Bm.exe has a significant number of command line options. To view a full listing, type `bm.exe ?` at the command prompt.

Using bm.exe, you can deploy, undeploy, and view a history of changes. To deploy your definition file, at the command prompt, enter this command:
```
Bm.exe <path to your configuration file>\<configuration file name>
```

> **NOTE**
>
> Bm.exe requires the .xls extension on configuration files in order to locate them successfully.

Chapter 6 - Business Activity Monitoring

Assuming you have selected RTA for your BAM definition, after you execute bm.exe you should see a screen similar to Figure 6.14.

```
Command Prompt
bm.exe undeploy #{change number} [BAM Configuration file]
bm.exe {add|remove} <BAM view name> <NT account> [BAM Configuration file]
bm.exe list <BAM view name> [BAM Configuration file]
bm.exe listchanges [BAM Configuration file]

- OPTIONS -
help: Displays this help text.
dbsetup: Sets up primary import, star-schema and analysis databases.
deploy: Deploys BAM infrastructure.
undeploy: Undeploy BAM infrastructure.
          When "view" option is used, only views are undeployed.
          When "all" option is used, both views and activities are undeployed.
          When "#" option is used, undeploy all deployed by the change number.
add: add NT account to the role associated with specified view.
remove: remove NT account from the role associated with specified view.
list: list all NT accounts which have been added to the specified view.
listchanges: list all deployment and undeployment which have succeeded.

- PARAMETERS -
<BAM Definition file>:
BAM definition XML file or BAM Excel workbook file name.

[BAM Configuration file]:
Optional, default to BamConfiguration.xml at current directory if not provided.

<BAM view name>:
BAM View name.

<NT account>:
NT group or user account.

C:\Program Files\Microsoft BizTalk Server 2004\Tracking>bm deploy "c:\MyEntropy\
Projects\book\BTS_HC\BAM definition files\BAMBTSbook.xls"
Retrieving BAM Definition XML from Excel workbook ... Done!
Deploying PrimaryImportDatabase ... Done!
Deploying ArchivingDatabase ... Done!
Deploying DataMaintenanceDTS ... Done!
Updating connection strings in Excel workbook ... Done!
Saving live data copy of the Excel workbook to c:\MyEntropy\Projects\book\BTS_HC
\BAM definition files\BAMBTSbook_LiveData2.xls ... Done!

C:\Program Files\Microsoft BizTalk Server 2004\Tracking>_
```

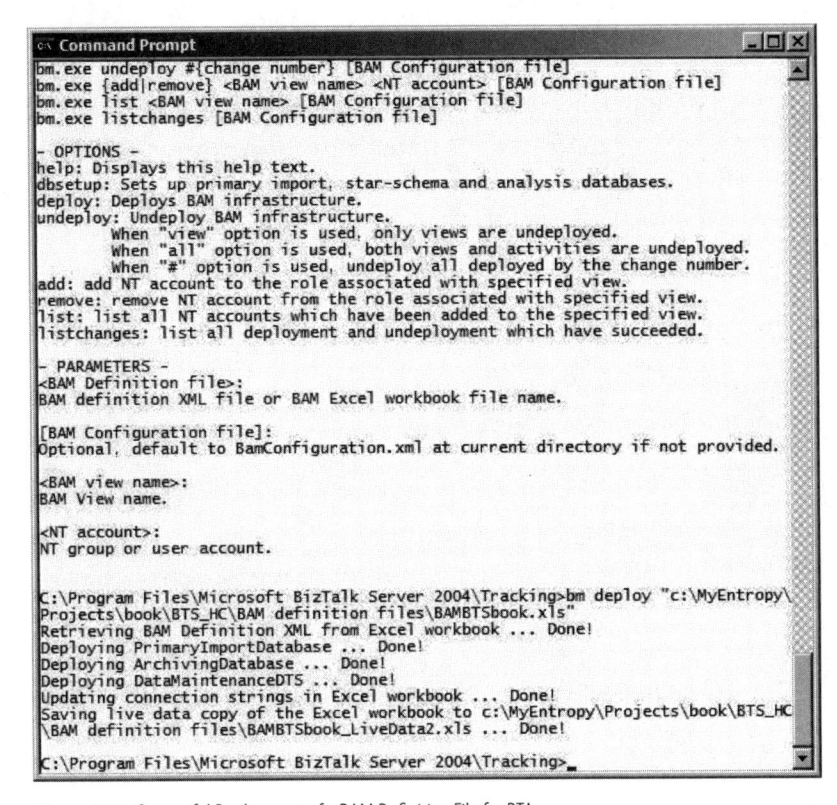

Figure 6.14: Successful Deployment of a BAM Definition File for RTA.

If you did not select RTA, the success message will have the following content:

```
Retrieving BAM Definition XML from Excel workbook ... Done!
Deploying PrimaryImportDatabase ... Done!
Deploying StarSchemaDatabase ... Done!
Deploying AnalysisDatabase ... Done!
Deploying ArchivingDatabase ... Done!
Deploying CubeUpdateDTS ... Done!
Deploying DataMaintenanceDTS ... Done!
Updating connection strings in Excel workbook ... Done!
Saving live data copy of the Excel workbook to c:\MyEntropy\Projects\book\BTS_HC\BAM
⮑definition files\BAMBTSbook_LiveData1.xls ... Done!
```

Regardless of your deployment option, a new file will be created in the same directory as your BAM definition file. This file will be named <BAM definition file name>_LiveData.xls. If a file already exists with the same name, it will append a number to the end. This is the file that will eventually be used by the business user.

The undeploy function of bm.exe can be very picky. If you don't have the original BAM definition file or you forgot to save changes under a different file name, you cannot use the bm undeploy <BAM definition filename> option. Instead, first type:

```
Bm listchanges.
```

This will give you a listing like this:

```
C:\Program Files\Microsoft BizTalk Server 2004\Tracking>bm listchanges
#1: Deploy ProNet_BAMViews.xls BamConfiguration.xml
        By HAL2004\BTS at 2/12/2004 11:34:52 PM (v3.0.4902.0)
        Activities: PatientTracking
        Views: HeadNurseView
#2: Deploy ProNet_BAMViews.xls BamConfiguration.xml
        By HAL2004\BTS at 2/13/2004 10:22:02 AM (v3.0.4902.0)
        Activities: EncounterTracking
        Views: AdminView
```

Note the number that precedes each deployment. Now, you can undeploy by the number associated with the view by typing

```
Bm undeploy #<the number associated with the definition>
```

This is a bit of a hack, and is not the cleanest approach, but it works.

Populating the BAM View and Tracking BAM Activities

After deploying the BAM definition, the BAM infrastructure is ready to receive data. The way that data is received by the BAM infrastructure is through the event bus. The event bus can be accessed in one of two ways: the API in the BAM Software Development Kit (SDK), or the orchestration layer.

Integration Using the BAM SDK

One of the ways that the BAM infrastructure can interact with external systems is via an API that ships standard with the product. This approach allows fine-grained, code-level control over how events are reported to the BAM event bus and also allows for events outside the scope of BizTalk to interact with the BAM infrastructure.

This technique can also be used to notify the BAM layer of events as they pass through a BizTalk pipeline component. This approach is relatively straightforward and is covered extensively in the product documentation. The focus of the remainder of this chapter will be on integration at the orchestration layer, since this leverages a much more code-free approach to building linkages between BizTalk Server and Business Activity Monitoring.

Integration at the Orchestration Layer with the Tracking Profile Editor

If the activities you need to monitor have been implemented as part of either one or multiple orchestrations, BizTalk has a set of tools which allow you build a code-free linkage to the BAM infrastructure. The Tracking Profile Editor (TPE) is a graphical design tool that allows you to tie business data and context data from an orchestration to specific business activities defined as part of a deployed BAM definition. By using the TPE, you can rapidly map data from promoted properties, distinguished fields, and context data, such as the start and/or end time of an event. Before using the TPE, make sure that you have deployed your BAM definition and any orchestrations that you need to work with. Once complete, open the TPE from the BizTalk Server 2004 program group.

The sole purpose of the TPE is to create a *tracking profile*. As depicted in Figure 6.15, the tracking profile binds the orchestration data to the BAM activities you defined in the BAM configuration file.

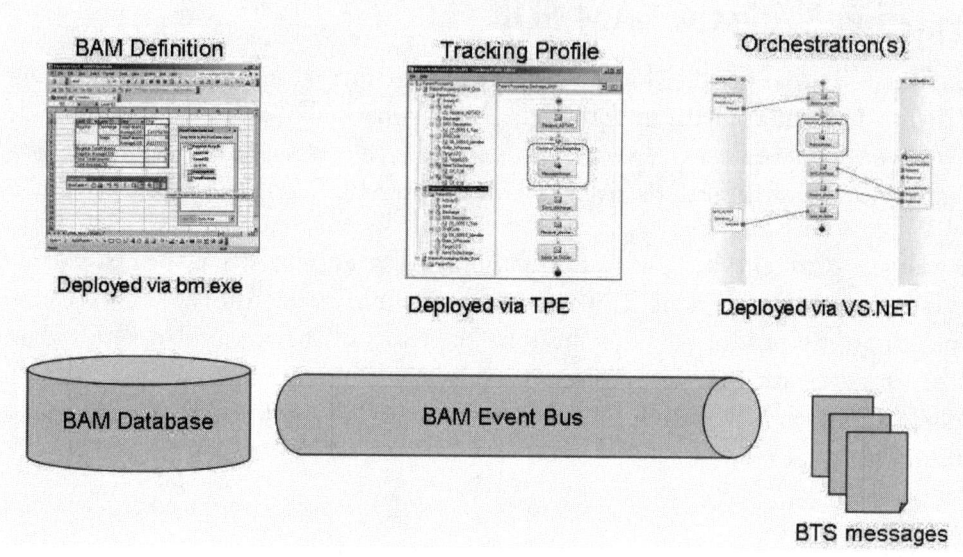

Figure 6.15: The Tracking Profile Binds the BAM Definition with One or More Orchestrations.

Creating A New Tracking Profile

Follow these steps to create a new tracking profile.

1. Open the TPE and select **File** ⇨ **New**. Figure 6.16 shows the dialog window that will appear. Select the assembly that contains the orchestration(s) that you would like to tie to the BAM definition. If your orchestration assembly does not appear, make sure it has been deployed.

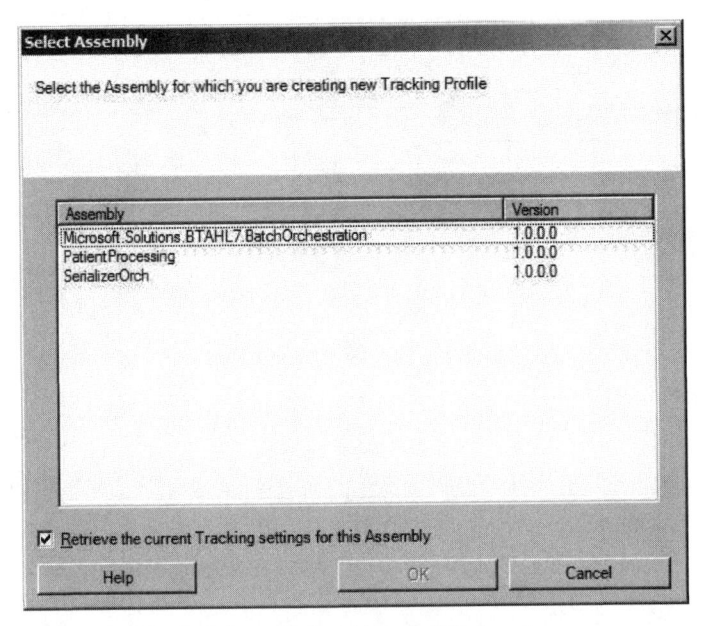

Figure 6.16: Select the Orchestration Assembly for the TPE to Import.

2. Click the **OK** button. All of the orchestrations contained in the assembly will be shown in the right-hand pane.

> **TIP**
>
> If you want to correlate multiple orchestrations in a BAM view and wish to use the TPE, make sure that all of the orchestrations are in the same assembly.

3. To tie your orchestration to a BAM definition, right-click one of the orchestrations and select **Import Activity Definition**. Figure 6.17 shows an activity definition being tied to an orchestration.

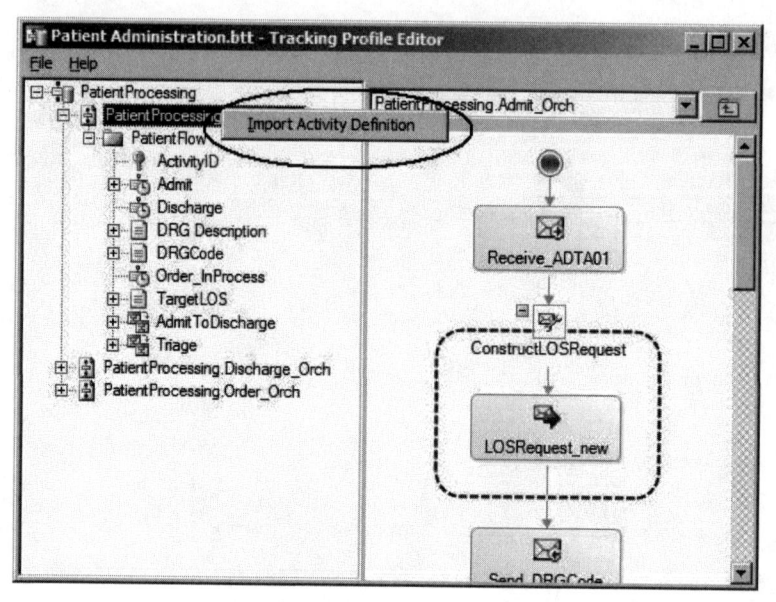

Figure 6.17: Importing a BAM Activity Definition into the TPE.

The activity definition is not the Excel spreadsheet itself, but an XML document that is created in the deployment process.

4. Navigate to the directory where you stored your BAM definition spreadsheet, and you should see an XML file in the same directory. Select this file and click the **OK** button. You will see a list of all of the BAM activities appear under each orchestration.

5. To map data fields to the BAM activity, right-click on a Message shape as shown in Figure 6.18, and select **Messages/Parts**. The screen shown in Figure 6.19 will appear in the main window of the TPE, allowing you to drill down into a message and view the schema associated with that step in the orchestration.

Chapter 6 - Business Activity Monitoring

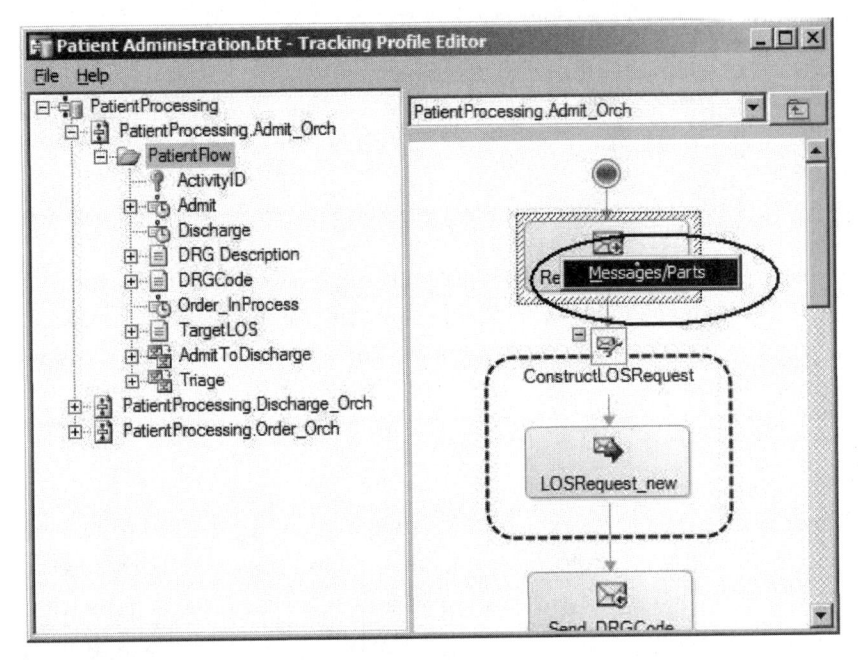

Figure 6.18: Selecting the Message to Inspect.

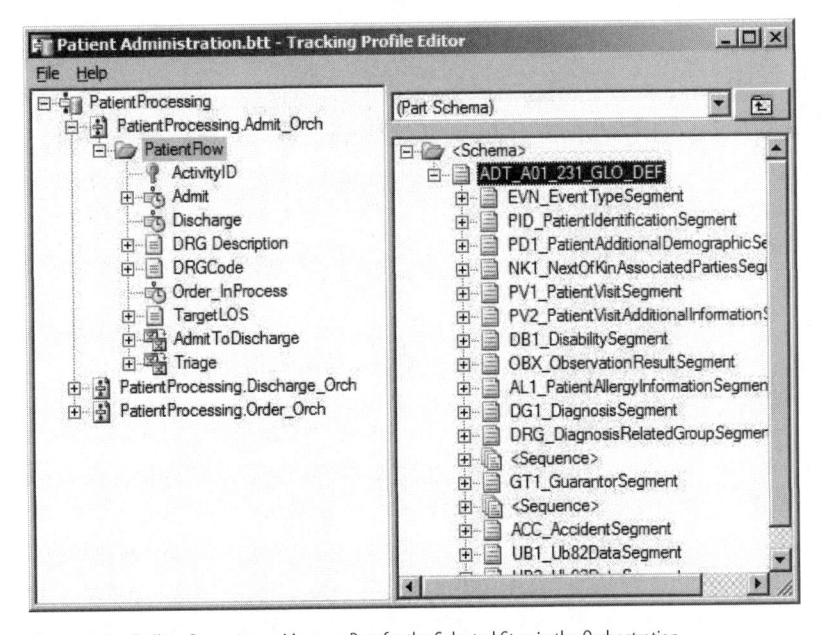

Figure 6.19: Drilling Down into a Message Part for the Selected Step in the Orchestration.

119

6. To map an element in this message to a business activity, simply drag and drop the data element from the left-hand pane to the business activity on the right.

> **TIP**
>
> **When working with HL7 data, the MSH segment will not be available in the TPE. Map these fields to a custom segment (often called a "ZSegment") if needed in a BAM view. For information on HL7 data and the MSH segment, see Chapter 7.**

7. You will notice that business activities that were configured as milestones appear in the list with a clock icon next to them. To populate these activities, select the orchestration step that is related to this activity, right-click on the activity, and select **Associate with end of selected action**.

Keep in mind that if you have multiple orchestrations being aggregated in a view, you will only populate milestone information for activities that occur within a particular orchestration.

For example, you would not populate the **Patient Discharged** milestone while working with the **PatientProcessing_Admit_Orch** orchestration in the TPE because that orchestration has no discharge activity. Instead, populate the milestone under the child elements listed under the **PatientProcessing_Discharge_Orch** orchestration where the **Patient Discharged** activity can be tied the appropriate step in the orchestration.

Aggregating Events with Continuation Tokens

The TPE also allows you to use *continuation tokens* to build relationships between orchestrations for the purpose of BAM reporting. A continuation token is a key that tells the BAM infrastructure that two disparate orchestrations are part of the same overall end-to-end process. In the TPE, you define the unique identifiers of the token (usually part of the message payload), which are composed of a composite or single field in the message itself. For example, if we have an admit process that is separate from a discharge process, we can link the two together under a continuation token defined by **patient ID** and **encounter ID**.

Chapter 6 - Business Activity Monitoring

Keep in mind that these orchestrations can operate completely independently of each other during runtime. Creating a continuation token only binds orchestrations together at the BAM layer, and this will not affect how messages are processed by the system.

Creating a Continuation

Use the following steps to create a continuation token between two orchestrations.

1. In the TPE, select the orchestration that happens first in the series. Right-click on the orchestration in the left-hand pane and select **New Continuation**, as shown in Figure 6.20. A new icon will appear in the tree structure as a child to the orchestration. Figure 6.20 shows the initiation of a continuation in the **Admit** orchestration, because it precedes the **Discharge** orchestration.

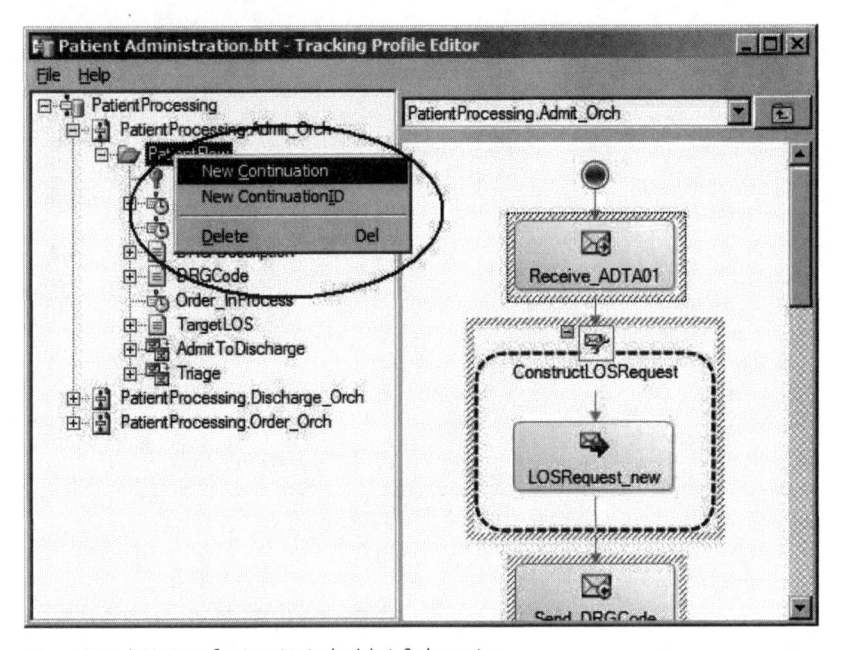

Figure 6.20: Initiating a Continuation in the Admit Orchestration.

2. Switch to the Schema view in the TPE (shown in Figure 6.19). Identify the data elements that will relate this message to other messages in this business process, and drag them to the continuation node in the selected orchestration (in the left-hand pane). For example, you might drag and drop a claim number and subscriber SSN to this field if it uniquely identifies the process.

3. Select the orchestration that will follow the orchestration from Step 1. Right-click in the left-hand pane and select **New ContinuationID**, as shown in Figure 6.21. You will see a key icon appear in the tree structure below the orchestration.

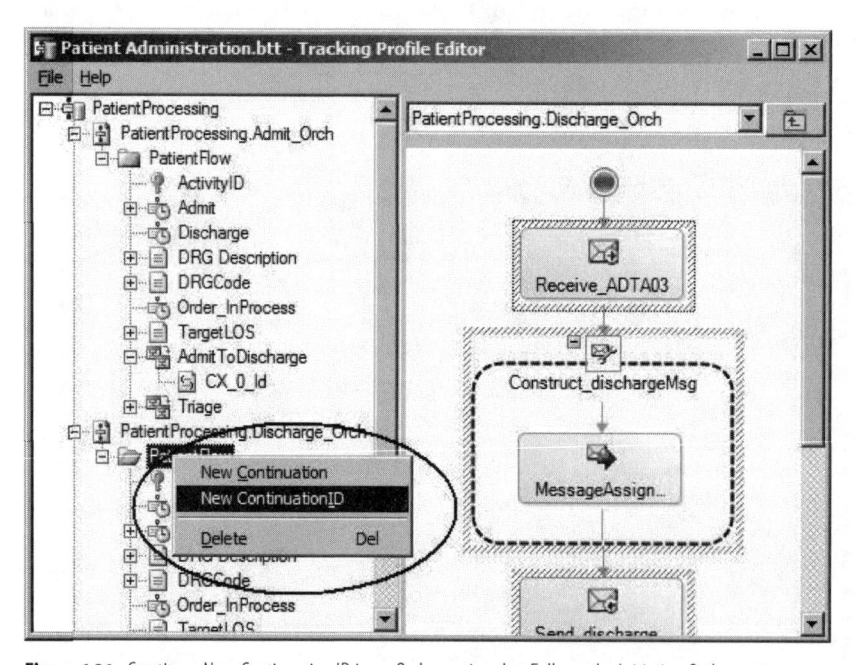

Figure 6.21: Creating a New Continuation ID in an Orchestration that Follows the Initiating Orchestration.

4. Map data fields from the messages available in this orchestration that correspond to the ones you selected in the continuation initiator. These elements can appear in totally different message structures; only the values of the elements matter.

Once you have completed the steps above, any messages that have a match between data that appears in a continuation initiator and any subsequent continuation followers will be correlated at the BAM layer. This will allow you to calculate, for example, end-to-end processing time for a business process that spans multiple orchestrations.

Deploying the Tracking Profile

Once all data, context information, and continuations have been mapped, you are ready to deploy the tracking profile. To do this, select **Deploy** from the **File** menu in the TPE. A confirmation message box will appear.

Viewing BAM Activities

To view the reporting on the activities you have defined, open the spreadsheet created by the bm.exe tool called <BAM definition file name>_LiveData.xls. When the spreadsheet workbook opens, you will see a pivot table similar to Figure 6.22.

DRGDescription	Data	Total
CARPAL TUNNEL RELEASE	AverageLOS	0
	AverageRecovery	0
	AvgTriagewait	0.000493248
	LOSTarget	2.2
	NumberofPatients	1
DEMO BROKEN ARM	AverageLOS	0.005106674
	AverageRecovery	0
	AvgTriagewait	0
	LOSTarget	0.0001
	NumberofPatients	2
Total AverageLOS		0.00340445
Total AverageRecovery		0
Total AvgTriagewait		0.000164416
Total LOSTarget		0.7334
Total NumberofPatients		3

Figure 6.22: BAM Pivot Table Populated Using Real-Time Aggregation (RTA).

> **TIP**
>
> If you have not run any data through the system and attempt to open the LiveData spreadsheet, you will get an error that the pivot table could not be refreshed. To resolve this, simply run some data through the orchestrations and the error message will disappear.

Your pivot table information will initially load with the most current data. However, if you leave the worksheet open, you can refresh the data by clicking on the red exclamation point in the pivot table toolbar, as shown in Figure 6.23.

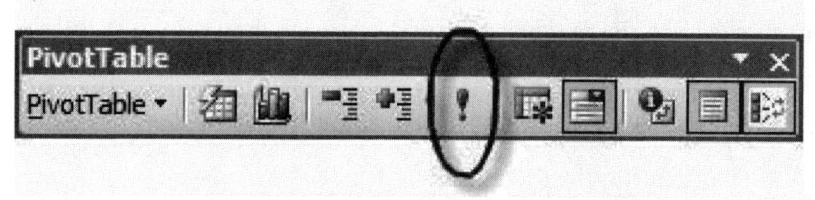

Figure 6.23: Refresh Button in Pivot Table Toolbar.

Charts and Graphs

A powerful way to display the information that is tracked by BAM is through a chart or graph. Since BAM's user experience is based on Excel pivot tables, you can easily build charts and graphs using Excel's native functionality in these areas. Figure 6.24 shows a simple chart of a hospital's workload, grouped by Diagnostics Related Group (DRG) and average wait times.

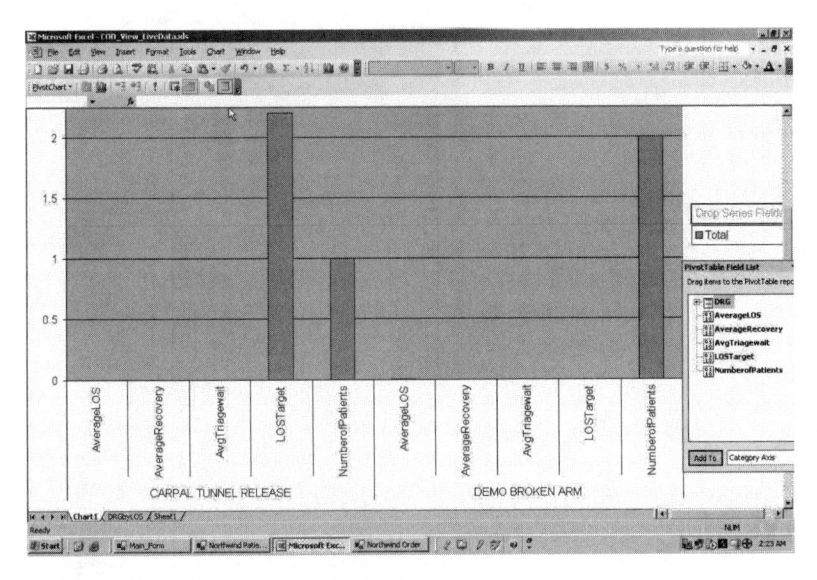

Figure 6.24: Charts Built on Data from the BAM Infrastructure.

Summary

With the coming of BizTalk Server 2004, easily implemented business activity monitoring has moved past the hype and into reality. By leveraging Excel, business users have a familiar user experience where they can define what kind of metrics they want to track. They can view the data and build their own charts and reports from that data.

By using BizTalk orchestration, you can implement business activity monitoring without having to write any code. For more complex scenarios, including activities that take place outside the scope of BizTalk, an API is available for code-driven interaction with the BAM infrastructure.

Microsoft has built a solid, easy-to-implement BAM solution that can be rapidly implemented. Deploying BAM is not technically challenging, so take the time to implement a few scenarios. Once deployed, BAM crystallizes the value of having an integration strategy and platform.

> **Did you know?**
>
> Microsoft's BizTalk home page contains a tremendous amount of useful information, including updated documentation for Business Activity Monitoring. Example implementation scenarios for Business Activity Monitoring are also available from the site.
>
> The BizTalk home page can be accessed at `www.microsoft.com/biztalk`.

Part II

HL7 and HIPAA

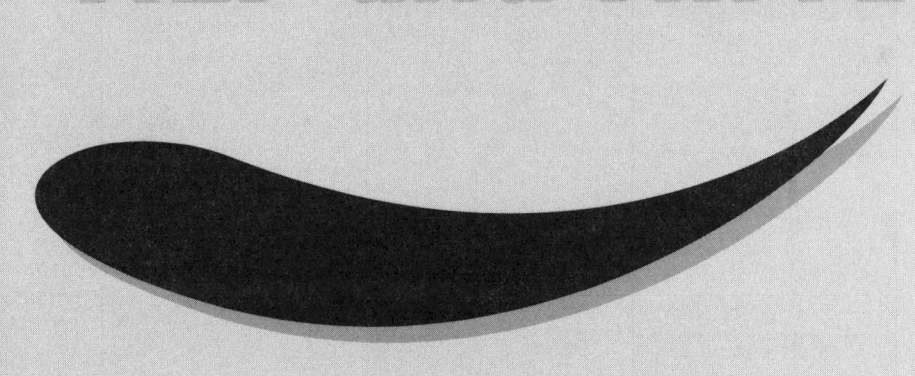

Chapter 7

Integration Challenges of HL7 Processing

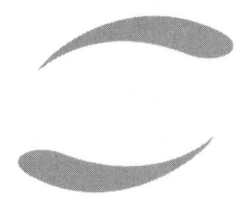

Rationalizing the data that is transferred between disparate systems so that it can be easily understood and interpreted is absolutely necessary in any integration scenario. From the beginning, data rationalization has best been accomplished by the creation of standards. Once defined, a standard serves as common ground for otherwise separate and distinct systems. While each system remains individually charged with translating the common data language into its own language, all systems can now communicate without having to understand each system's "native tongue." Figure 7.1 below illustrates how communication between two separate systems is facilitated by a common data language.

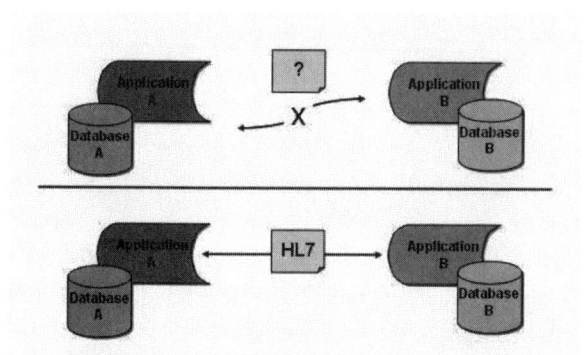

Figure 7.1: Data Standards Like HL7 Enable Separate Applications to Share Data.

While helpful, data standards alone do not completely address industry-specific integration needs. In addition to providing a common language, industry use eventually dictates associated practices centered around how the data will be communicated and processed—rules of engagement, if you will.

On a high level, the rules of engagement between internal applications that are sharing data are different than when data must be shared externally between organizations. For internal applications, the concern is in automating and monitoring the continuous movement of data between applications. However, for external applications, data must be processed securely between organizations that are often using asynchronous transports like HTTP over unreliable networks like the Internet, with data errors being communicated automatically.

In healthcare, specific practices have evolved that dictate how data is shared. Internally, data is typically shared in an HL7 format. Externally, data is traditionally shared in an EDI format, and more recently in the United States, in a HIPAA-mandated format. For information on the HIPAA standard, see Chapters 9 and 10.

HL7 Overview

HL7, as an acronym, is an anomaly because it stands for both a data structure and the organization charged with defining its structure. Officially meaning Health Level Seven, it takes its name from seventh level (the application level) of the Open Systems Interconnection (OSI) interoperability stack defined by the International Organization for Standardization (ISO), which develops standards for data networking. Figure 7.2 shows the OSI healthcare model with HL7 at the seventh level.

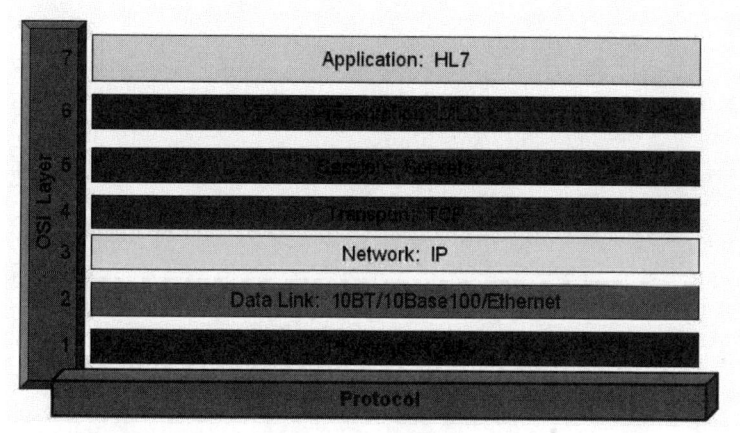

Figure 7.2: Healthcare OSI Model, with HL7 at Seventh Level.

Interoperability was the primary concern of HL7's founders in 1987, when they were first looking at ways to rationalize the data that needed to be exchanged between systems in a healthcare organization. Each department in a healthcare organization typically uses a system that has specific features to meet the department's needs. Following a "best of breed" approach, individual departments typically use a system that has unique features to support its specific data needs. These are referred to as Line of Business (LOB) applications. It is not uncommon for a single organization to have 30 to 50 LOB applications, each working independently from the others.

The challenge, however, is that patient information must be shared between all of the individual Line of Business applications in a single healthcare organization. As illustrated in Figure 7.3 below, the only way to share patient data between systems (absent a common data language) was to create a point-to-point interface between the two systems. Since multiple systems share not only basic patient information, but also share specific LOB information directly, point-to-point, individually coded interfaces are hugely inefficient, more difficult to manage, and ultimately more expensive to maintain over the long run.

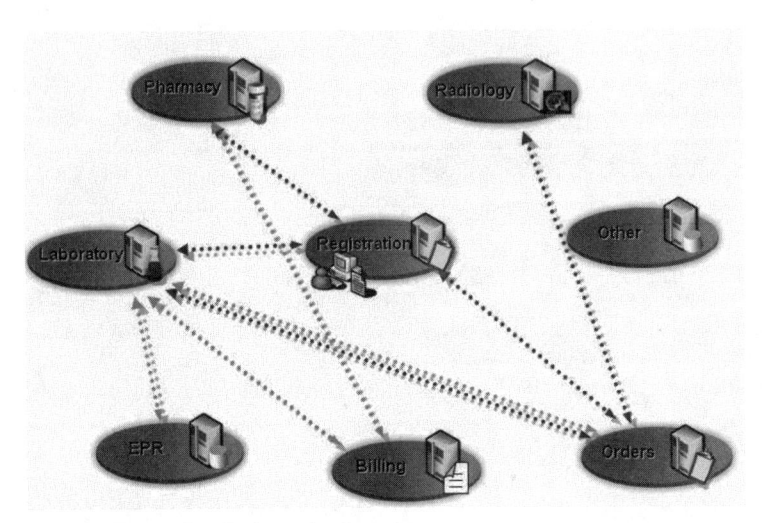

Figure 7.3: Point-to-Point Application Interfaces.

This is where a data standard comes in. Systems can more readily exchange data when they are all using a common data language. By using a common data language, each line of business application is charged with accepting and creating data in the common format. Once done, interfaces can be shared and an integration tool such as BizTalk Server 2004 can be used to eliminate the point-to-point coding that used to be required, as shown in Figure 7.4 below.

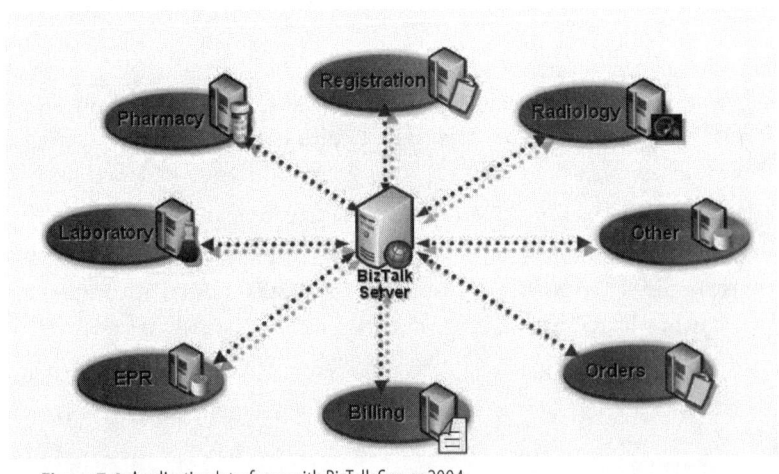

Figure 7.4: Application Interfaces with BizTalk Server 2004.

Created to be a framework for building integrated health systems, HL7 is an ANSI-approved data standard that is used today in 27 countries worldwide, including over 90% of hospitals in the United States. Simply referred to as "HL7," there are actually nine versions of the data standard in use today, eight that have been formally approved, and one that is soon to be approved but is already in use in a few countries outside of the United States, as shown in Table 7.1.

Version	Date Approved
2.0	September 1988
2.0D	October 1988
2.1	March 1990
2.2	December 1994
2.3	May 1997
2.3.1	April 1999
2.4	October 2000
2.5	September 2003
3.0	TBD

Table 7.1: HL7 Versions.

The HL7 Organization

The HL7 standard was created by volunteers working together as part of Health Level Seven, Inc., which is an ANSI-approved standards organization. Founded in 1987, the HL7 organization includes members from healthcare providers, vendors and consultants. While the organization initially defined the HL7 data standard, its mission goes beyond simple message definition.

The HL7 organization's official mandate is to provide standards for the exchange, management, and integration of data that support clinical patient care and the management, delivery, and evaluation of healthcare services. Their goal was to create flexible and cost-effective approaches to standards, guidelines, methodologies, and related services directed towards the interoperability between health information systems.

As designed, the HL7 standard offers many benefits. On a basic level, the standard enables information exchange between computer applications developed by different vendors. Thus, healthcare providers can continue their reliance on best of breed applications, because the standard allows the disparate systems to work together. By rationalizing data between systems, HL7 reduces the labor and time associated with point-to-point interfaces and allows for the integration of health information over time and across delivery systems.

HL7 is an evolving standard that is designed to allow for new functionality while supporting legacy implementations. Unlike traditional data standards that contain specific rules for the creation and placement of data, the HL7 standard is really more of a specification. It serves as a functional guideline for creating HL7 messages.

The specification is identified through two primary structure types: flat file delimited data (as seen in all of the Version 2.x standards) and XML-encoded data, as defined in Version 2.XML (which for all intents and purposes is Version 2.x data encoded as XML) and Version 3.

As discussed further in this chapter, a limitation of the 2.x versions is that they serve as an information model for message content only. The standard does not contain encoding information. Version 3 constitutes the first real modeling effort by the HL7 organization. HL7 Version 3 data is encoded as XML and contains several layers of data modeling information before the actual message content. In addition, it contains much more rigid message structure rules. Because of this, Version 3 messages are not backwards compatible with the 2.x versions. As of this writing, it is estimated that Version 3 will not be fully implemented world-wide for a few years to come.

NOTE

Today, Version 2.x data is the most widely used, with Versions 2.2 and 2.3 being used in the majority of implementations today. For that reason, this chapter focuses on Version 2.x. For more information on the Version 2.XML and Version 3 standard, visit `www.hl7.org`**.**

A Brief Look at the 2.x Message Structure

The 2.x versions of the HL7 specification define data that is "pipe and hat" delimited, meaning that data components are encoded with "|" and "^" symbols. Figure 7.5 shows a sample Version 2.x HL7 message.

```
MSH|^~\&|ERADMIT|MAIN|BILLING|MAIN|200309241123||ADT^A01|9876|P^I|2.3.1
EVN|A01|200309241123
PID||88888^^^PRIMARY|99999^^^LAB|U6123456|SMITH^HARRY^T|Babasafa|19610521|MALE||123
    CENTER STREET^METROLOLIS^IL^60016^USA^HOME||(555)123-
    4567||ENGLISH|M|CATHOLIC|3|444-55-6666|555555555^IL
PV1|1|E|EMERGENCYROOM^ROOM3^BED1|E|||4421^WELBY^MARCUS^^^^
AL1|1||^PENICILLIN||PRODUCES HIVES~RASH~LOSS OF APPETITE
AL1|2||^DOG HAIR|RESPIRATORY DISTRESS
```

Figure 7.5: Sample Version 2.x HL7 Data.

Version 2.x messages are designed around message segments. Groups can be thought of as simply a collection of segments or other groups. The major component in an HL7 message is therefore the *segment*. A segment is a delimited line of data that contains data relevant to one specific use in the message. For example, patient identification information is in one segment while any patient allergies are defined in another segment. Each segment is then composed of data fields. Each data field can have one or more components. Each component may have sub-components. A hierarchical representation is shown in Figure 7.6.

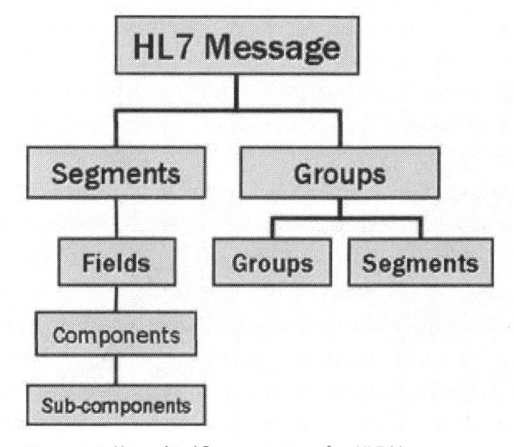

Figure 7.6: Hierarchical Representation of an HL7 Message.

Figure 7.7 shows an example of what an actual patient identification (PID) segment might look like as part of an HL7 message.

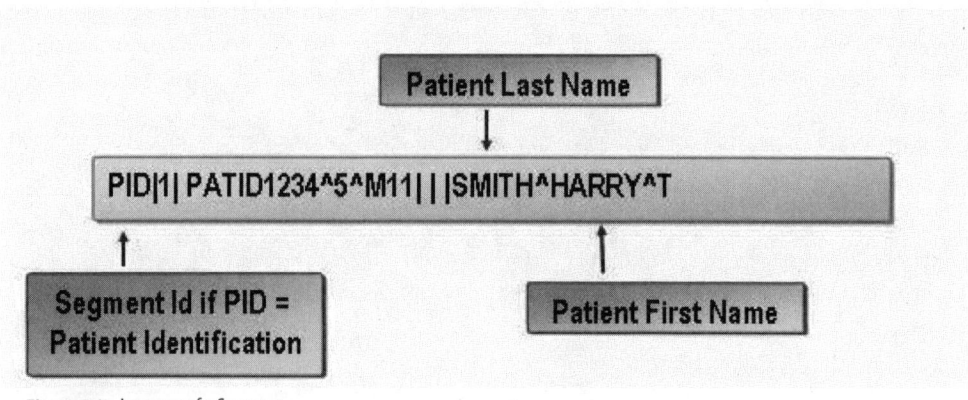

Figure 7.7: Anatomy of a Segment.

Every message is composed of a header segment, the **MSH** Segment, and then the message body, composed of multiple segments, some individually and some in looping structures. Segments take on meaning based on their placement in the message. The standard defines whether they may only appear one time, or whether they are allowed to repeat. When they repeat, their physical placement indicates the data relevance. For instance, as seen in Figure 7.8, if a patient has two allergies, there will be two AL1 (allergy) segments.

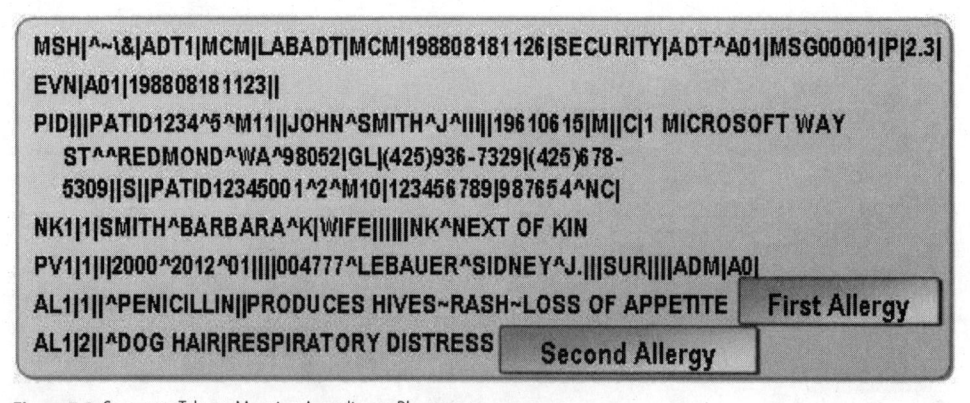

```
MSH|^~\&|ADT1|MCM|LABADT|MCM|198808181126|SECURITY|ADT^A01|MSG00001|P|2.3|
EVN|A01|198808181123||
PID|||PATID1234^5^M11||JOHN^SMITH^J^III||19610615|M||C|1 MICROSOFT WAY
    ST^^REDMOND^WA^98052|GL|(425)936-7329|(425)678-
    5309||S||PATID12345001^2^M10|123456789|987654^NC|
NK1|1|SMITH^BARBARA^K|WIFE|||||NK^NEXT OF KIN
PV1|1||2000^2012^01||||004777^LEBAUER^SIDNEY^J.|||SUR||||ADM|A0|
AL1|1||^PENICILLIN||PRODUCES HIVES~RASH~LOSS OF APPETITE     First Allergy
AL1|2||^DOG HAIR|RESPIRATORY DISTRESS     Second Allergy
```

Figure 7.8: Segments Take on Meaning According to Placement.

Basically, segments are logical groupings of data fields. They are identified by a 3-character Segment ID that starts each segment. Each segment is then terminated by a carriage return or a carriage return/line feed. The data fields in a segment are typically separated by a "|" symbol and are referred to by their position in a segment, such as PID.1 for the first field in the PID Segment. The components inside of a data field are separated by "^" symbols and can repeat. When they repeat, their values are separated by "~" symbols. The delimiter characters used for the component separator, field repeater, escape delimiter, and (rarely used) subcomponent delimiter are defined in the first field of the **MSH** Segment. All components with a data field are optional, because the standard specifies only data field optionality, and it does not address optionality in levels contained within the data field. Thus, if a data field is present, it can have optional components. Figure 7.9 shows a sample Version 2.x HL7 message with data fields highlighted to show the inclusion of optional components.

```
MSH|^~\&|ERADMIT|MAIN|BILLING|MAIN|200309241123||ADT^A01|9876|P^I|2.3.1
EVN|A01|200309241123   Date and Time of Admission    Patient Administration Message
                                                     Patient has been admitted
PID||88888^^^PRIMARY|99999^^^LAB|U6123456|SMITH^HARRY^T|Babasafa|196
   10521|MALE||123 CENTER
   STREET^METROLOLIS^IL^60016^USA^HOME||(555)123-     Attending Physician
   4567||ENGLISH|M|CATHOLIC|3|444-55-6666|555555555^IL Physician ID^Last^First
PV1|1|E|EMERGENCYROOM^ROOM3^BED1|E|||4421^WELBY^MARCUS^^^^
AL1|1||^PENICILLIN||PRODUCES HIVES~RASH~LOSS OF APPETITE
AL1|2||^DOG HAIR|RESPIRATORY DISTRESS
```

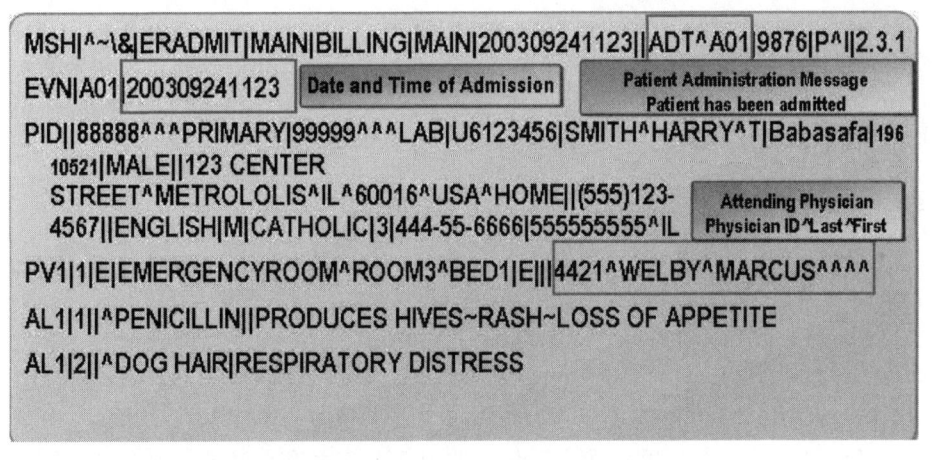

Figure 7.9: Sample Patient Administration Message.

What makes the structure particularly challenging from an integration perspective is that messages can contain segments that are not part of the standard. Called *locally-defined segments*, they are identified by a Segment ID code beginning with a "Z." Thus, they are commonly referred to as *Z Segments*, and they allow added flexibility. The standard dictates that they always appear at the end of a message, after all standard-defined segments. However, industry use often finds them scattered throughout a message structure.

The structure is complex and can be difficult to interpret. While there are some mandatory components to every message type, the specification allows for backwards compatibility between versions through optional components. Basically, changing mandatory field values across versions is possible by making previously mandatory fields optional. This results in redundant field values and opens the standard up for individual interpretation, essentially enabling different flavors of the same message type. In the end, the specification serves primarily as a detailing of message components loosely built around a suggested framework.

In a lot of ways, the Version 2.x HL7 specification is similar to what happens when you build a custom motorcycle. The specification serves as the general plan for building the motorcycle. With the plan, you know what parts you absolutely must have, like an engine and gas tank, along with what parts are simply nice to have, like a radio. You also know that certain parts on the motorcycle will have to go together in a certain way. Beyond that, however, the rest is up to individual interpretation. You are left to decide on the quality and specifications of the parts you are using, as well as what extra parts you want to include. With Version 2.x HL7, the specification is your motorcycle plan which provides the common framework to work within. Actual HL7 integration scenarios are as diverse and unique as custom-built motorcycles.

Version 3, Anyone?

A limitation of the 2.x versions is that they serve as an information model for message content only. The standard does not contain encoding information. Version 3 constitutes the first real modeling effort by the HL7 organization. HL7 Version 3 data is encoded as XML and contains several layers of data modeling information before the actual message content (Figure 7.10 shows a sample Version 3.0 message). In addition, Version 3 contains much more rigid message structure rules than are found in 2.x. Because of this, Version 3 messages are not backwards compatible with the 2.x versions.

```xml
- <ns0:POLB_IN002121 xmlns:ns0="urn:hl7-org:v3">
    <ns0:creationTime value="2004-11-03T15:59:08"
    <ns0:acceptAckCode code="AL" />
    <ns0:versionId>V3R1B6</ns0:versionId>
  - <ns0:controlActProcess>
    - <ns0:subject>
      - <ns0:ObservationOrder classCode="OBS" mood
          type="Observation">
        <ns0:id root="2.16.840.1.113883.9876.34$
          extension="187963" />
        <ns0:effectiveTime value="200401291745"
      - <ns0:recordTarget>
        - <ns0:patient>
          - <ns0:patientLivingSubject>
            - <ns0:Person classCode="PSN"
                determinerCode="INSTANCE">
              - <ns0:name>
```

Figure 7.10: Sample Version 3 HL7 Data.

Because it is so different from the versions currently in use in the majority of healthcare organizations, it may be some time before HL7 Version 3 is widely adopted. However, Version 3 has many benefits that make ultimate mainstream adoption highly likely. Because backwards compatibility is not possible, Version 3 contains stricter structural rules, moving it from a specification to more of a true standard. The standard uses a Reference Information Model (RIM) to add meaning to the data in addition to the encoding that is inherently part of the XML structure. Ultimately, this should provide for easier interfaces since it limits the amount of individual interpretation that is currently required in the 2.x versions.

Because HL7 Version 3 has not been formally adopted as of this writing, the rest of this chapter will focus on the 2.x versions of HL7.

Even without the rigidness that Version 3 offers, the 2.x versions of HL7 serve the original purpose of enabling interoperability between healthcare applications. Serving as a framework for negotiation between applications, the standard enables the sharing of patient information by not only defining data content but by establishing transport and acknowledgement protocols.

Why Is HL7 Processing Special?

With HL7 processing, data flows between applications in individual messages. A single message relates to a single individual. Messages are referred to by a three character code related to the type of information the message is relaying. For example, messages containing patient administrative information use the code "ADT," while a message being used to order a medical procedure is defined by the code "ORM."

The assumption is that an event in the real world of healthcare creates the need for a message to be shared between two or more systems. This event is called a *trigger event*. Trigger events include changes in a patient's status from being admitted to being discharged, the ordering of a procedure, or the return of lab results. Trigger events are identified by a unique three character code. For example, the code "A01" would be used for a patient admission message, while the code "A03" indicates that the patient is being discharged.

Messages are used to ensure that all concerned applications in the facility are aware of the services being rendered to each patient. A new message will be generated each time the patient changes state in the facility. Thus, messages are referred to by the type of message, such as a patient administration message or an order message. They are further categorized by trigger event code, such as an A01 patient administration message, which indicates that the new administrative information in the message is that the patient was admitted to the facility. Since both codes are relevant, they will be encoded into the message header to describe the type of information contained in the message. They are generally referred to in the same fashion, so a patient administration message concerning a patient's admission would be referred to as an ADT^A01 message, where ADT is the message type and A01 is the trigger event code.

The challenge with this model is that a single patient will have many messages generated during a single visit, or stay, at the health facility. Each message is either broadcast from one system to all other clinical systems, as with patient administration messages, or it is directed to a specific application, as in the case of the ordering of a medical procedure. This translates to a high amount of continuous data flow between systems.

A Look at a Sample Data Flow

Let's take a look at the message flow generated from a common scenario, as illustrated in Figure 7.11 below. Our patient, Harry Smith, enters the emergency room with a broken arm. Harry is registered into the hospital information system (HIS). The HIS application broadcasts a patient administration message with an event code of A04 to all other hospital applications with Harry's information so that he has access to services. Depending on the size of the facility, the message could be routed to as many as 30 to 50 concerned applications.

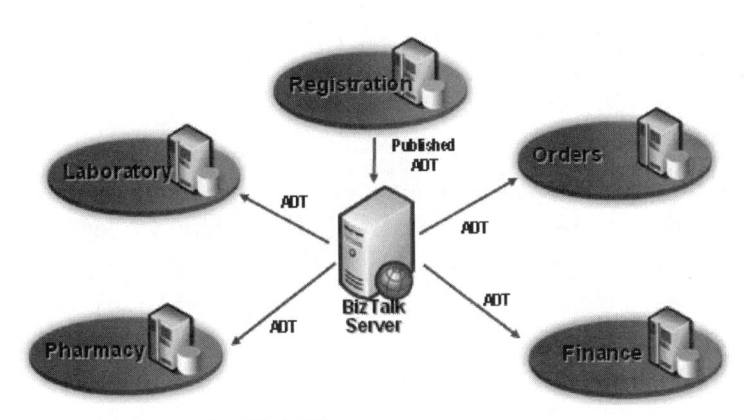

Figure 7.11: Broadcast of an ADT^A04 Message.

Harry needs an x-ray, so the doctor enters an order into the Order System, which then sends an order message (ORM^O01) to the Radiology System. When the results are ready, Radiology sends them to the Order System via an ORU^R01 message. Based on the x-ray results, Harry needs surgery and so will be admitted to the hospital. The surgical order will go out as a new ORM^O01, but this may need to go to multiple systems, each concerned with some aspect of the services Harry will need for his surgery. Additionally, an ADT^A01 message will be broadcast from the HIS system to all hospital applications that received the original ADT^A04 message to indicate the change in Harry's status from being registered to being admitted. Figure 7.12 illustrates the amount of individual messages that will flow between four systems based on our simple scenario.

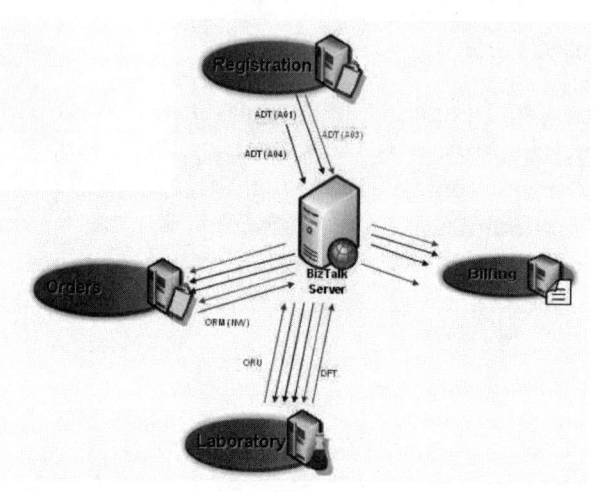

Figure 7.12: Message Flow Complexity.

During Harry's stay in the hospital, messages will be generated for procedures he needs, their results, and all services he receives, including changes to his physical location within the facility. Some of these messages will be sent directly to a single concerned application, as was the case between the Order and Radiology systems. However, most messages will need to go to more than one application. For example, the HIS and Billing systems will most likely monitor every message generated concerning Harry. Ultimately, Harry will be discharged via an ADT^A03 message going from the HIS system to all hospital applications.

Integration Challenges

The integration challenge raised by this continuous data flow per patient is in minimizing the amount of connections linking applications like spaghetti strings, and in guaranteeing the delivery of each message. Additionally, to speed processing, messages are usually streamed using TCP/IP rather than being transferred in a file format. This streamed data contains certain control characters to indicate the beginning and end of the data stream, following the Minimum Lower Layer Protocol (MLLP) that is defined in the OSI interoperability model shown in Figure 7.2. Streaming data between systems is commonly referred to as MLLP transport. Any HL7 integration scenario must include the ability to process data presented via MLLP transport. Finally, a good deal of HL7 processing today still takes place in batches, rather than in real-time. Any HL7 integration solution must contain the ability to handle both types of processing.

Spaghetti, Anyone?

BizTalk provides the necessary first step to minimizing the amount of spaghetti strings involved in the message flow through its publish/subscribe model. With BizTalk, each application is configured to route its messages through BizTalk. Separately, each application creates subscriptions within BizTalk for the message types it is interested in. Thus, rather than coordinating multiple direct and indirect connections, you simply focus on one application at a time and configure its specific interaction with BizTalk.

Verified Delivery

By focusing on the application's needs when configuring an interface in BizTalk, you are also able to address the second integration challenge—that of guaranteeing the delivery of each message. As discussed in Chapter 3, the difference between an *adapter* and an *accelerator* is that an accelerator brings with it pre-built functionality necessary to address industry-specific needs. In the case of HL7 processing, an industry-specific need is the ability to automatically acknowledge messages as they are received. The HL7 Accelerator for BizTalk provides just this ability. The accelerator brings with it an easy to use user interface for acknowledgment configuration, as shown in Figure 7.13. The details of configuring acknowledgments are discussed in greater detail in Chapter 8.

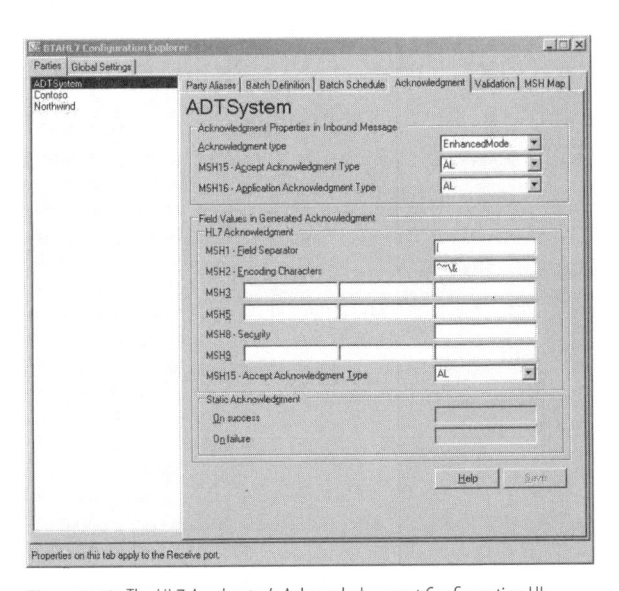

Figure 7.13: The HL7 Accelerator's Acknowledgement Configuration UI.

You Say MLP, I Say MLLP

The interchangeable terms Minimum Layer Protocol (MLP) and Minimum Lower Level Protocol (MLLP) both refer to the method of transferring data between applications quickly and inexpensively. Given the multitude of messages generated by a single patient, think of the sheer volume of messages that move each day in a healthcare facility. To write each message to a file would be an expensive drain on system resources. A less I/O-intrusive approach is to avoid the file layer and transfer the data via TCP/IP.

When data is streamed, special control characters are assigned to the beginning and end of the stream to indicate break points, as shown in Figure 7.14. The BizTalk Accelerator for HL7 accommodates this transfer protocol by including an MLLP adapter. Think of this adapter as providing the necessary information for BizTalk to pick up and separate the individual messages contained in the TCP/IP data stream so that they can be received or sent via BizTalk's messaging services.

<VT> HL7 Message Content   <FS> <CR>

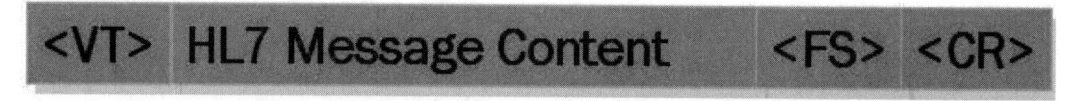

Figure 7.14: Message Start and Stop Characters Are Placed Around HL7 Messages Being Processed Via MLLP, with a Data Stream Terminating Character.

Real-Time? But We Save Resources by Batch Processing...

Batch processing is a common need with HL7 processing. Although officially designed for real-time message processing, BizTalk provides batch processing configuration through a convenient user interface, thanks to the addition of the BizTalk Accelerator for HL7, as shown in Figure 7.15. Through this interface, you can configure what messages are included in a batch as well as schedule batch run cycles. When a batch of messages is delivered to the BizTalk engine, each individual message will be separately validated, routed, and acknowledged.

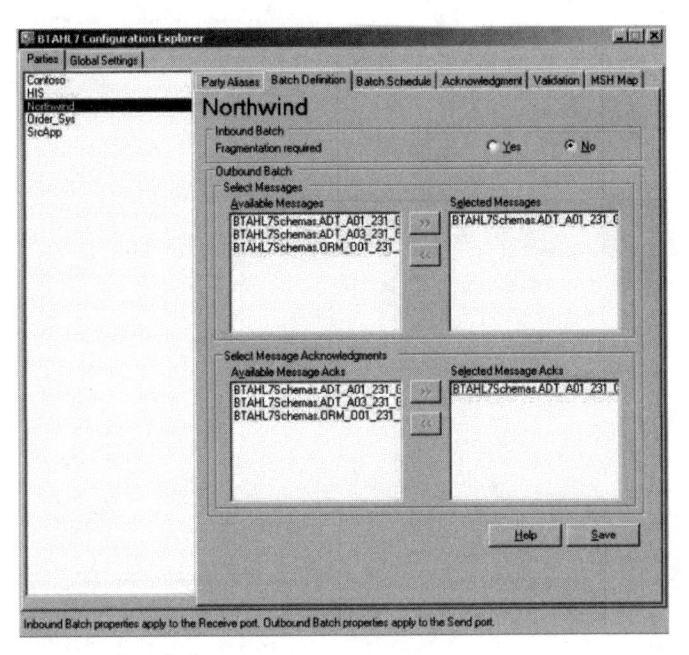

Figure 7.15: Batch Configuration.

Summary

The HL7 data standard insists that high volumes of data must be accommodated through automatic routing and acknowledgement. Further, data will often be transferred using a TCP/IP socket. The BizTalk Accelerator for HL7 was created to provide a solution to the challenges raised by these healthcare-specific processing needs.

> **Did you know?**
>
> You don't need to be a member of the HL7 organization to download the HL7 standards.
>
> Simply visit `http://www.HL7.org` and select HL7 Standards under the Resources column on the home page.

Chapter 8

The HL7 Accelerator for BizTalk Server 2004

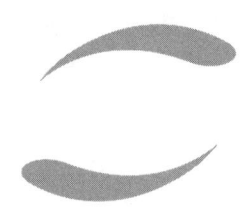

As a messaging standard, the HL7 message structure is a complex flat-file, delimited format. Luckily, BizTalk Server can take a complex message and represent the same data in XML. Not only is this more portable in terms of reuse and programmability, but it also makes the data much more readable by humans. All data that flows through BizTalk Server is internally represented as XML. This makes doing internal validation easier because it is based on schemas, and also simplifies data mapping via XSLT. The trick is to provide a means for BizTalk Server to convert the data from its native format to XML. BizTalk facilitates this conversion by parsing the data via disassembler (DASM) components within a BizTalk receive pipeline. When you need to then go from XML to flat-file format, a send pipeline is required. Pipelines leverage predefined schemas (such as the ones provided by the BizTalk Accelerator for HL7) to create and validate these messages.

The BizTalk Accelerator for HL7 (BTAHL7) simplifies the process of developing integrated HL7 solutions by adding key components and enhancements to the basic BizTalk platform. Included in the accelerator are more than 1,300 HL7 schemas for 2.1 through 2.4 message types, send and receive pipelines that leverage those schemas, a new adapter to support MLLP, as well as an additional tool, the BTAHL7 Configuration Editor, provided for easy acknowledgment and batch processing configuration. In this chapter, we'll look at the added functionality introduced by the accelerator and examine how to use these new tools.

The HL7 Schema

BizTalk uses XML Schema Definition (XSD) schemas (a W3C standard) to describe message formats. As discussed in Chapter 6, regardless of the data format you are processing, you must associate the data with a schema if you want BizTalk to validate it. The BizTalk Accelerator for HL7 comes with 1,300 predefined schemas to match every 2.x (2.1 through 2.4) message type. These schemas were generated from an Access database provided by the HL7 organization, so they are considered "official" definitions. For users that have access to the database, the accelerator includes the option to install the tool that was used to generate these schemas.

However, as we've seen previously, when it comes to a version 2.x message, you rarely see an "official" message. Rather, individual interpretations of messages abound. To accommodate this reality without adding a deafening amount of complexity to the schema, the data fields, segments, and tables identifying looping structures are defined in a separate schema file for each version to serve almost as a version-specific dictionary. Figure 8.1 shows a sample set of version-specific dictionary schemas.

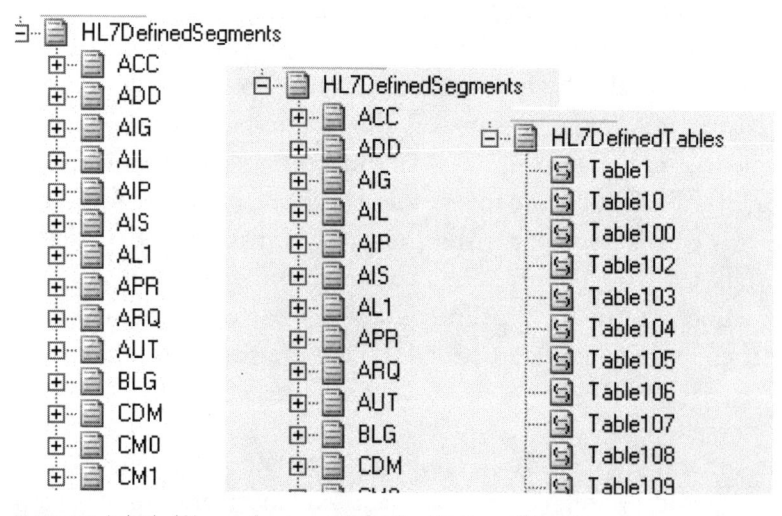

Figure 8.1: Individual Message Components Defined in a "Dictionary" Schema.

The HL7 Accelerator comes with individual message schemas for each message type, as seen in Figure 8.2. These individual message schemas depict the necessary message structure. Message schemas then reference the dictionary schemas for common individual definitions. You can think of this as the same way a Visual Studio .NET project may reference external assemblies to access classes. In fact, a BizTalk project follows the same reference rules as any object-orientated development project in Visual Studio .NET.

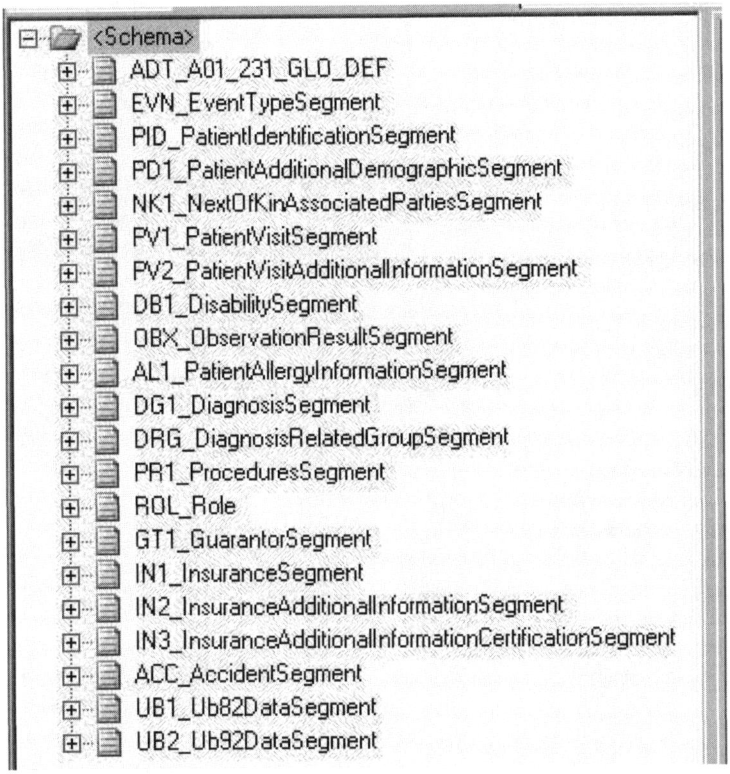

```
<Schema>
    ADT_A01_231_GLO_DEF
    EVN_EventTypeSegment
    PID_PatientIdentificationSegment
    PD1_PatientAdditionalDemographicSegment
    NK1_NextOfKinAssociatedPartiesSegment
    PV1_PatientVisitSegment
    PV2_PatientVisitAdditionalInformationSegment
    DB1_DisabilitySegment
    OBX_ObservationResultSegment
    AL1_PatientAllergyInformationSegment
    DG1_DiagnosisSegment
    DRG_DiagnosisRelatedGroupSegment
    PR1_ProceduresSegment
    ROL_Role
    GT1_GuarantorSegment
    IN1_InsuranceSegment
    IN2_InsuranceAdditionalInformationSegment
    IN3_InsuranceAdditionalInformationCertificationSegment
    ACC_AccidentSegment
    UB1_Ub82DataSegment
    UB2_Ub92DataSegment
```

Figure 8.2: Message Schema Depicting the Message Structure and Referencing Dictionary Schema for Individual Definitions.

The benefit of this definitional separation is that message structures can be both globally and locally altered from the official standard. If the user wishes to alter the definition of a segment or data field for every message that the user processes, the alteration would take place in the definitional schema. If the user wishes to only vary from the standard for that particular message type, the change can be made locally in the message schema. The benefit of this definitional separation is that the message schema appears to be less complex, and is thus easier to work with inside of the mapping tool.

Because of the backwards compatibility rules, the version 2.4 **MSH** Segment and acknowledgment (ACK) structures are appropriate for all prior versions. Regardless of the specific HL7 version you are processing, you will always have an **MSH** Segment and the engine will auto-generate acknowledgements. For this reason, separate schemas have been provided for the **MSH** Segment and for HL7 acknowledgements in a version 2.4 format. Figure 8.3 shows the **MSH** Segment schema.

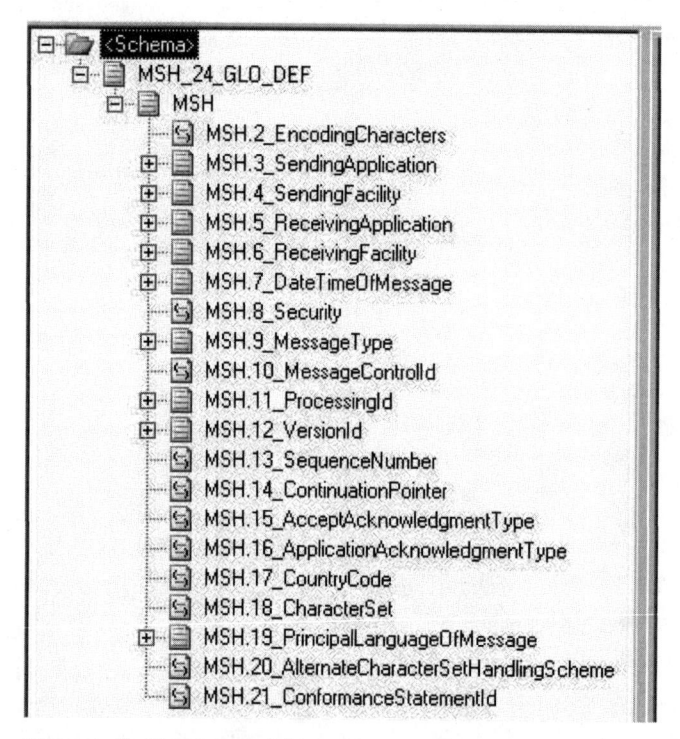

Figure 8.3: The Message Header Schema.

How you deploy and work with these different schemas is discussed later in this chapter.

The BTAHL7 Receive Pipeline

Receive pipelines provide a sequential set of stages to prepare data before it is published into the BizTalk message database. In the case of version 2.x HL7 data, the data must be parsed from its flat-file, delimited structure into an XML structure. The BTAHL7 Receive Pipeline, shown in Figure 8.4, contains its own disassembler component (DASM) that reads the **MSH** Segment to determine the message type and version. Based on this information, it then looks to the configuration database to locate the appropriate message schema that defines the message.

Armed with the schema that defines the structure, the data is then parsed, or disassembled, from its delimited structure and converted into XML for use by the BizTalk engine. As the data is disassembled, it is validated against the message schema. This parsing occurs within the disassembler component of the pipeline. The HL7 Disassembler is alternately referred to as the HL7 Disassembler or the HL7 DASM. Unlike the default flat-file DASM provided by BizTalk Server, the HL7 DASM does not require that a schema be specified per pipeline. Rather, the parser is able to determine which message schema to use to validate the message by reading the message type and version indicator fields in the **MSH** Segment.

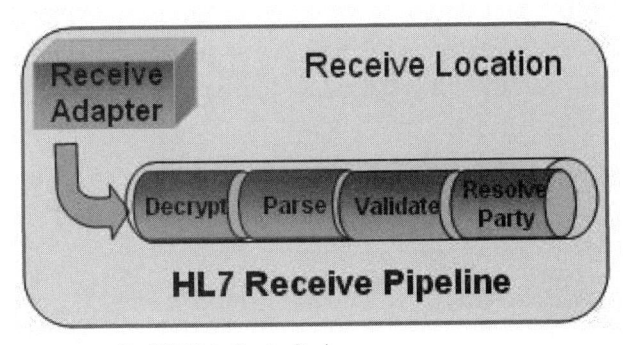

Figure 8.4: The BTAHL7 2.x Receive Pipeline.

The HL7 Disassembler provides the following functionality:

- Syntactic validation

- Dynamic delimiter validation

- Field validation

- Handles escape sequences
- Handles conditional optionality
- Handles defined and undefined or unexpected Z segments
- Ignores unexpected segments at the end of an instance
- Selects appropriate schema validation

Once the message is validated, the DASM also creates the appropriate acknowledgement(s) of the message. More than one acknowledgement may be created, depending on the acknowledgement level that was configured for the party sending the original message. As discussed later in this chapter, the DASM will create system and application level message acknowledgements. These are created after validation by the HL7 DASM component and both the XML format of the message and acknowledgement are then published to the BizTalk message box where they will remain until picked up by subscribing systems.

Working with the BTAHL7 Receive Pipeline

The BTAHL7 Receive Pipeline is automatically deployed when you install the BizTalk Accelerator for HL7. You need do nothing special to use the pipeline in your HL7 receive locations. Figure 8.5 shows a receive location utilizing the HL7 Receive Pipeline.

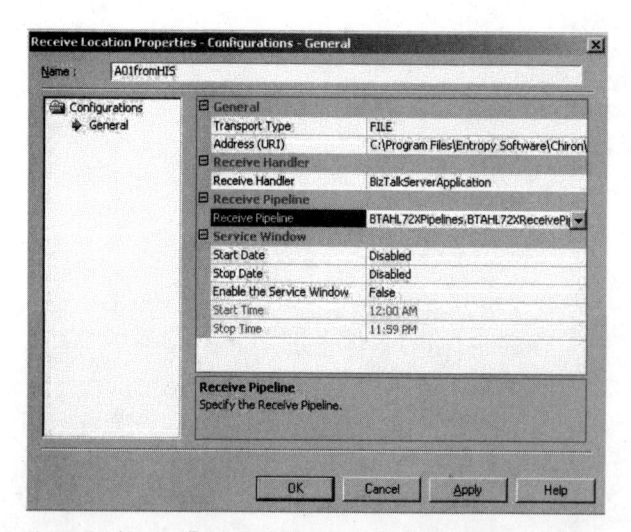

Figure 8.5: Locations Receiving HL7 Data Must Use the BTAHL7 Receive Pipeline.

However, functionally speaking, the BTAHL7 Receive Pipeline is simply a custom BizTalk pipeline, as seen in Figure 8.6. Because of this, you can re-use the HL7 DASM within your own custom pipelines and add additional components before or after the HL7 DASM stage. This is useful if you need to preprocess the data before publication to the message box.

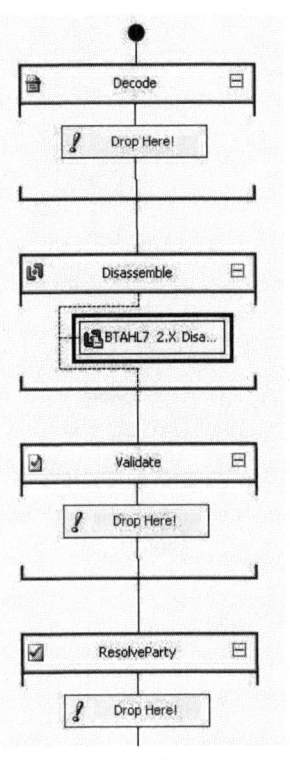

Figure 8.6: The BTAHL7 Receive Pipeline.

The stage at which you place the custom component will depend on what you need to do to the data. If you want to split or decrypt the message for some reason before it is parsed into XML, place the component before the HL7 DASM, in the Decode stage of the pipeline. If you want to split or alter the data after it has been converted to XML but before publishing, place the component after the HL7 DASM, in the Validation or Resolve Party stages.

In addition to customizing the BTAHL7 Receive Pipeline, you can use it to process non-HL7 data. A benefit of this would be the ability to have the non-HL7 data acknowledged automatically.

The HL7 DASM component uses the **MSH** Segment to determine the message type (MSH.9) and version (MSH.12). The HL7 Schemas are named according to message type and version as well, such as ADT_A01_23_GLO_DEF.xsd. In Figure 8.7, **ADT_A01** identifies the message type, matching the MSH.9, and **2.3.1** identifies version 2.3.1, matching the MSH.12.

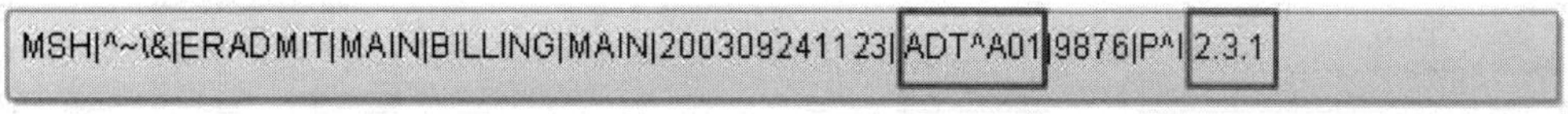

```
MSH|^~\&|ERADMIT|MAIN|BILLING|MAIN|200309241123|ADT^A01|9876|P^|2.3.1
```

Figure 8.7: The BTAHL7 DASM Uses the MSH Segment to Determine Which Schema to Use to Parse Data.

To process non-HL7 data, you simply need to preprocess the data to add an **MSH** Segment to the beginning of the data. This can be accomplished by adding a custom component to the BTAHL7 Receive Pipeline before the HL7 DASM component. If you create MSH formatting and place identifiers in the MSH.9 and MSH.12 fields that match the naming conventions of the HL7 message schema, the HL7 DASM will validate the non-HL7 data contained after the **MSH** Segment according to your data-specific schema. The HL7 DASM will then parse the data into BizTalk's internal XML format and create an HL7 acknowledgement for the engine to process. Just as with HL7 data, different levels of acknowledgements can be configured. Based on the set configuration, one or more ACKs may be published to the message box. We'll examine how to configure and use these acknowledgments later in the chapter.

> **NOTE**
>
> If you do not wish to receive an HL7-formatted acknowledgement from BizTalk, you can always write a map to convert the auto-generated acknowledgement into a format you specify, since HL7 Acknowledgement schemas are installed along with the message schema. Refer to Chapter 4 for a discussion of mapping options.

The BTAHL7 Send Pipeline

Similar to the BTAHL7 Receive Pipeline, the BTAHL7 Send Pipeline uses the HL7 message schema to assemble (or serialize) and validate the structure of the data to a delimited flat-file before it is sent to subscribing systems. Essentially, the HL7 Assembler (HL7 ASM) takes the XML document from the BizTalk message box and returns an HL7-encoded message.

Working with the BTAHL7 Send Pipeline

As with the BTAHL7 Receive Pipeline, the BTAHL7 Send Pipeline is automatically deployed upon installation of the BizTalk Accelerator for HL7. The BTAHL7 Send Pipeline will be used in all send port definitions that are subscribing to HL7 data and require HL7 output. Figure 8.8 shows a send port configured to use the BTAHL7 Send Pipeline.

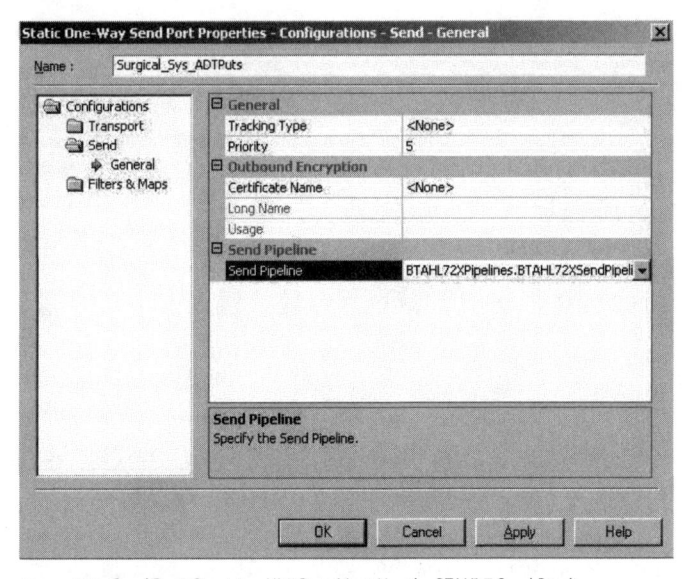

Figure 8.8: Send Ports Receiving HL7 Data Must Use the BTAHL7 Send Pipeline.

As with the BTAHL7 Receive Pipeline, the HL7 ASM can be re-used in your own custom send pipelines. A component added before the assembly stage will affect the data while it is still in its XML form, while a component added afterwards will occur once the data has already been serialized into an HL7-encoded message. Figure 8.9 shows the BTHL7 Send Pipeline.

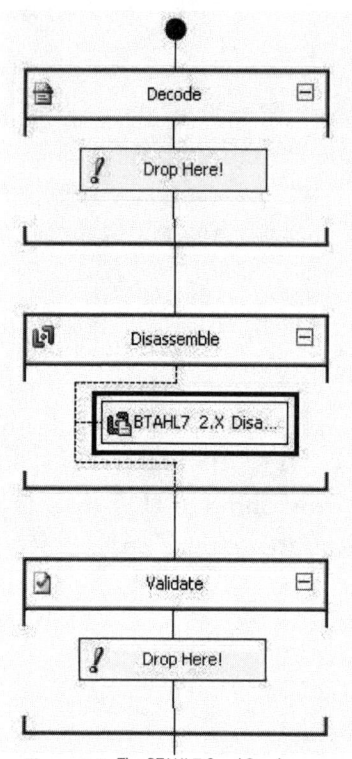

Figure 8.9: The BTAHL7 Send Pipeline.

Working with the HL7 Schema in BizTalk

Now that you know how the HL7 pipelines use the HL7 schema to parse and serialize data; we need to look at the process of configuring the schema for use by BizTalk. BizTalk Server can only access objects that have been deployed to the configuration database. That means that all relevant schemas, the MSH and ACK, as well as the dictionary and message types of schema, must be deployed in order for the DASM and ASM to construct and validate messages.

To understand what needs to be deployed, let's look at the provided schemas. Starting with the premise that both definitional and message structure schemas are provided for each version of HL7, we know that we will need to deploy both of these schema types. Because the message structure schemas rely on the definitional schemas, we need

Chapter 8 - The HL7 Accelerator for BizTalk Server 2004

to make sure that the message structure schemas have the appropriate reference to the definitional schemas once deployed. Additionally, we will need to deploy the schemas that define the **MSH** Segment and acknowledgements (ACK).

> **NOTE**
>
> The necessary deployment steps are defined below, but please refer to the End to End Tutorial found in BizTalk Accelerator for HL7 Help documentation for detailed guide to this process.

Deploying the Project Containing MSH and ACK Schemas

The first step in configuring BizTalk to process HL7 data is to deploy the message header and acknowledgement schemas. In the Solution Explorer in Visual Studio .NET, open the predefined BizTalk HL7 project called BTAHL7V2XCommon Project. This contains the MSH and ACK schemas, as shown in Figure 8.10.

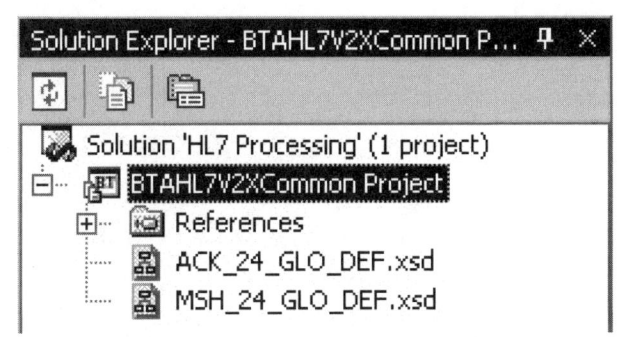

Figure 8.10: BTAHL7V2XCommon Project Contains Schemas for the MSH Segment and HL7 Acknowledgments.

Create and set a required Assembly Key (.snk) file, and deploy the project. Deploying this project is a one-time step that is necessary for all of your HL7 processing, because the message header and acknowledgement schemas are now available in the configuration database.

Deploying the Version-Specific Definitional Schemas

Definitional schemas are provided for each of the 2.x versions in predefined BizTalk projects by version. You will need to deploy the appropriate project for the HL7 version you are processing, according to the following steps.

1. In the Solution Explorer, add an existing HL7 project. The projects are located under HL7 schema projects and are identified as BTAHL7V231Common Project, where the "V231" indicates the version number. When this project opens in the Solution Explorer, notice that three schemas are included in the project, as shown in Figure 8.11: **datatypes_231.xsd**, **segments_231.xsd**, and **tablevalues_231.xsd**.

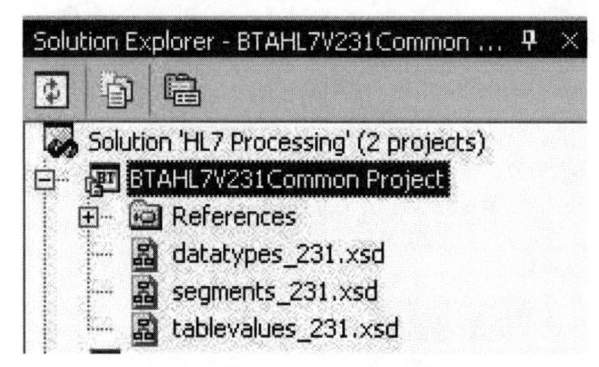

Figure 8.11: BTAHL7V231Common Project Contains the Definitional Schema Referred to by All Version 2.31 Message Schemas.

2. After applying the necessary Assembly Key (.snk) file, deploy the project. Deploying this project is a one-time step that is necessary for all of your Version 2.31 processing, because the definitional schemas referenced by all Version 2.31 schemas are now available in the configuration database.

Deploying Specific Message Schemas

Once the header, acknowledgement, and version-specific definitional schemas are deployed, you will configure and deploy message-specific schemas as necessary for your HL7 processing.

Chapter 8 - The HL7 Accelerator for BizTalk Server 2004

1. In the Solution Explorer, add an empty HL7 project. In this project, you will add a reference to the previously deployed project containing the definitional schemas for the message version you are processing. For instance, if you are processing a Version 2.31 ADT message, you would reference the Version2.31CommonProject you just deployed, as shown in Figure 8.12.

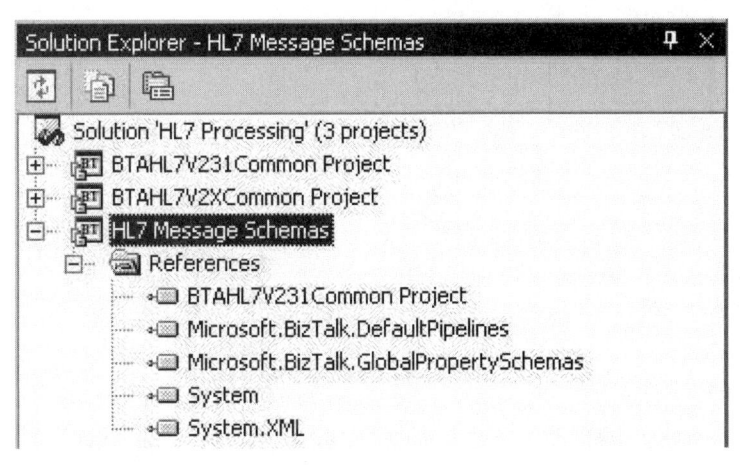

Figure 8.12: Reference the Version-Specific Definitional Schema in Your HL7 Message Project.

2. Once the reference is added, you will add a message schema to this project for each message type you are processing. To do this, add a new item to the project by selecting **Schemas** under the **BTAHL7 Items** category in the **Add New Item** dialog box. The **HL7 Schema Selector** dialog box, as seen in Figure 8.13 below, will open. In the **HL7 Schema Selector** dialog box, select the version and message type you are interested in. For example, if you are processing a Version 2.31 ADT^A01 message, choose 2.31 for the **Version**, ADT for **Message Type**, and A01 for **Trigger Event**. This will add the message definition schema to your project.

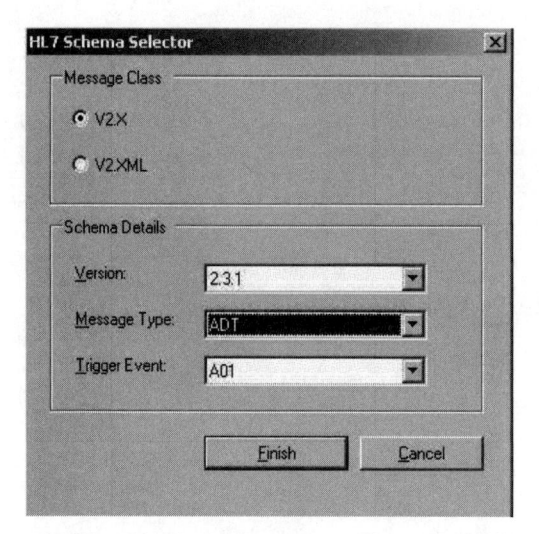

Figure 8.13: Select Version, Message Type, and Trigger Event Code to Add a Message Definition Schema.

3. Once you have added all of the message schemas you are interested in, apply the necessary Assembly Key (.snk) file and deploy this project. The schemas you added will be those that you will reference and use in your maps and orchestrations.

> **NOTE**
>
> For ease of maintenance, it is a recommended practice to deploy your message schemas separately from maps and orchestrations.

Configuring Acknowledgements

The HL7 Receive Pipeline automatically generates HL7 acknowledgements. However, if you do not configure BizTalk appropriately, the acknowledgements will sit unprocessed in the message box.

The accelerator makes use of Party definitions to associate acknowledgements to sending applications. A *Party* is the means through which BizTalk uniquely identifies a sending application by associating the sending application's identifier with the specific acknowledgement and batching configurations desired for that application. Once a Party has been defined, the BTAHL7 Configuration Editor is used to configure the type and format of the acknowledgements sent to that Party. You need to add a Party for each application that sends data to BizTalk. The Party definition must contain the value that the particular application places in the MSH.3 field in the message header, as that is how the parser matches the data to the Party definitions.

As shown in Figure 8.14, Parties are defined and configured in the BizTalk Explorer, according to the following procedure.

1. Add a Party by right-clicking the **Parties** tab under your configuration database in BizTalk Explorer and selecting **Add New Party**.

2. Give the Party a name that is relevant to your processing.

3. In the **Alias** column, enter the value that occurs in the MSH.3 field in the message header. Under the **Ports** tab, select the send port that is subscribing to the acknowledgement going to this application.

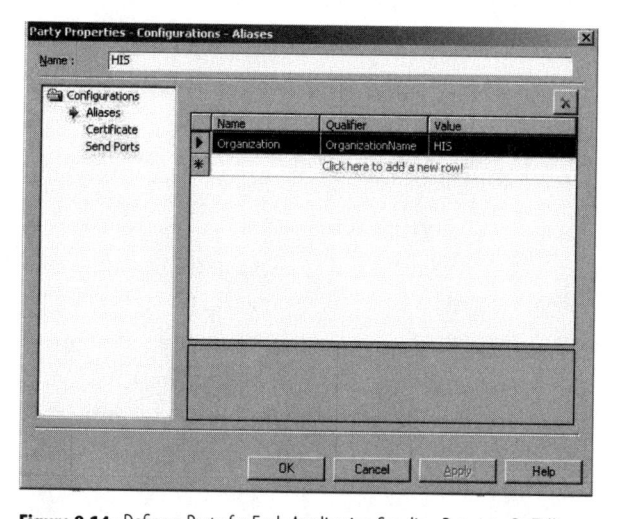

Figure 8.14: Define a Party for Each Application Sending Data into BizTalk.

4. Once the Party has been defined, you can configure the acknowledgements going to this Party in the BTAHL7 Configuration Explorer (accessed via the **Start** menu), as shown in Figure 8.15. You can define the level of acknowledgement you want to generate, along with any changes you would like to make to the **MSH** Segment in the acknowledgement.

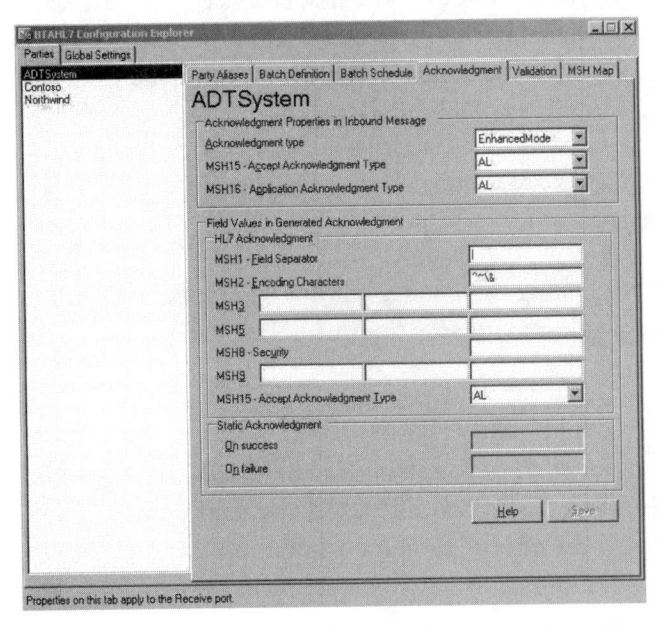

Figure 8.15: BTAHL7 Configuration Explorer.

Configuring Batch Processing

You also use the BTAHL7 Configuration Explorer to control batch content and scheduling. Batch processing is configured on a Party basis. Once your Parties are defined in BizTalk Explorer, you can control their batch schedules in the BTAHL7 Configuration Explorer. For each Party, you define the messages and acknowledgements to include in each batch, and then use the **Batch Schedule** tab to control the batch schedule, as shown in Figure 8.16.

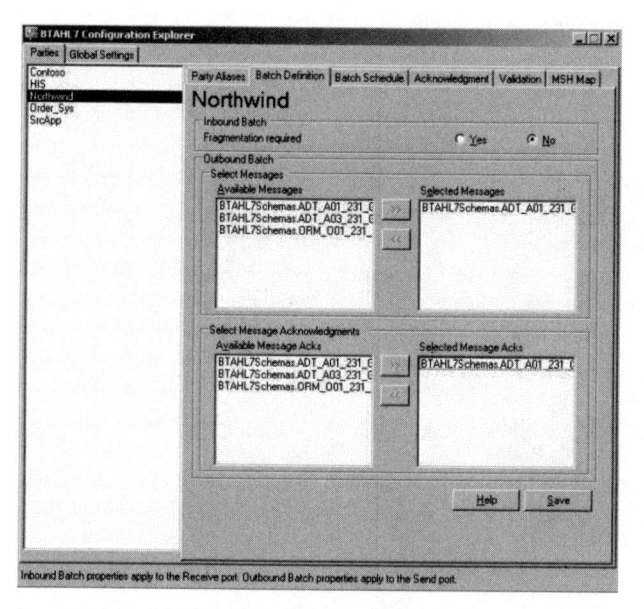

Figure 8.16: Batch Configuration is Available in BTAHL7 Configuration Explorer.

Configuring the MLLP Adapter

When processing data via TCP/IP using MLLP, the only extra step you need to take is to configure your receive location or send port to use the MLLP Adapter. The adapter is configurable as a one-way or two-way processor on the same socket, so you can receive a message and send an acknowledgement over the same socket. The choices are available in a handy user interface that is accessed through the URL settings in the receive location and send port configuration dialog boxes. Figure 8.17 shows the MLLP settings user interface accessed while configuring a receive location.

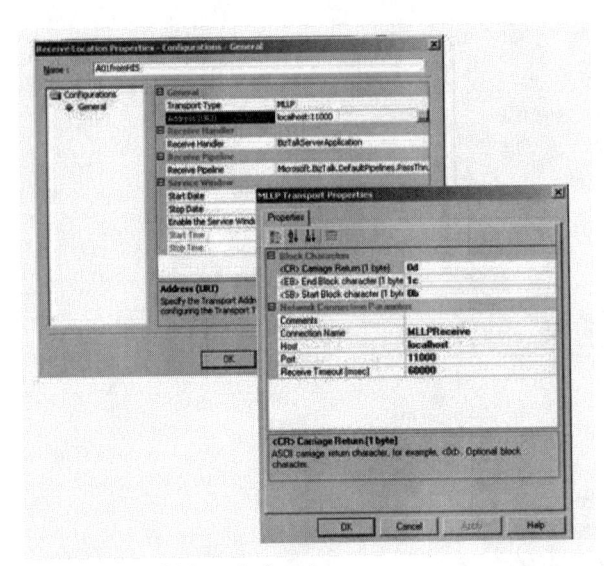

Figure 8.17: MLLP Adapter Configuration.

To receive data using MLLP, you will create a receive port and receive location through the BizTalk Explorer. In the **Receive Location** dialog box, select **MLLP** as the **Transport Type** and then click the browse buttons in the **Address (URI)** entry. This brings up a dialog box that allows you to configure the host and socket information along with the control characters that appear around the data. Once configured, you will select the HL7 Receive Pipeline to process the data.

To send data using MLLP, you will create a send port and use the HL7 Send Pipeline. As with the receive location, you will select **MLLP** as the **Transport Type** and bring up the configuration dialog box in the **Address (URI)** entry. This dialog box contains similar settings to the receive location dialog box and is used to configure the host and socket over which you are sending data.

Mapping HL7 Data

Although you need the BizTalk Accelerator for HL7 to process HL7 data correctly, it is important to remember that you have access to all the basic components of BizTalk as well. That means that you can send the data through maps or orchestrations as needed. Given the varied data structures of Line of Business Applications, the odds are that you will need to transform your HL7 data into a new shape or that you will need to create HL7 data from an old shape. You will use BizTalk maps to accomplish these tasks.

The BizTalk mapping tool allows for only a single input and output to a map. This translates to a single schema on the input and a single schema on the output. The schema you use for HL7 data is the message schema you deployed earlier in this chapter. That message schema defines the segment structure for only the body of the message. (Remember, the **MSH** Segment has its own schema.) Thus, when mapping HL7 data, you only have access to the body of the message. When mapping from HL7 data, this generally is not an issue because the body of the message contains everything in the message header segment except the sending and receiving system identifiers. However, when mapping to HL7, you will need to take some extra steps to assign an **MSH** Segment to the beginning of the message body that your map creates.

When mapping from HL7 data to a new format, you will use the HL7 message schema that matches your input data as the Data Source Schema. You then use a schema that defines your desired output as your Destination Schema. Once both are defined, you can drag and drop HL7 field components to the appropriate output element, using functoids to alter the data as necessary. Figure 8.18 below shows a map that is creating a non-HL7 format from HL7-formatted data.

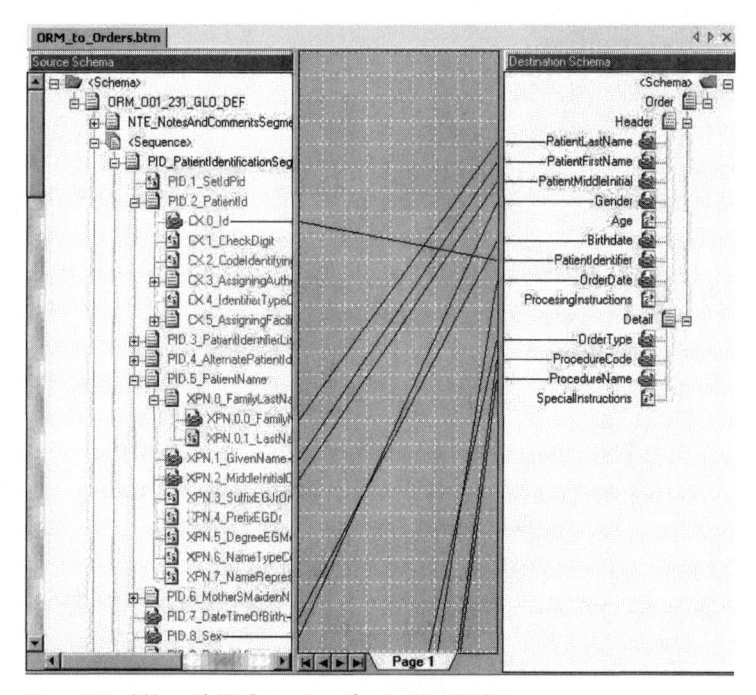

Figure 8.18: A Map with HL7 Data as Input Creating Non-HL7 Data.

Once the map is complete, you can test it before you deploy it, according to the following steps.

1. Open the properties window for the map and enter input data information. Indicate if you want BizTalk to validate the input to the map when it runs.

2. Right-click the map file in Solution Explorer and select **Test Map**, as shown in Figure 8.19. This will generate an output file that you can link to through the **Output** window in Visual Studio .NET.

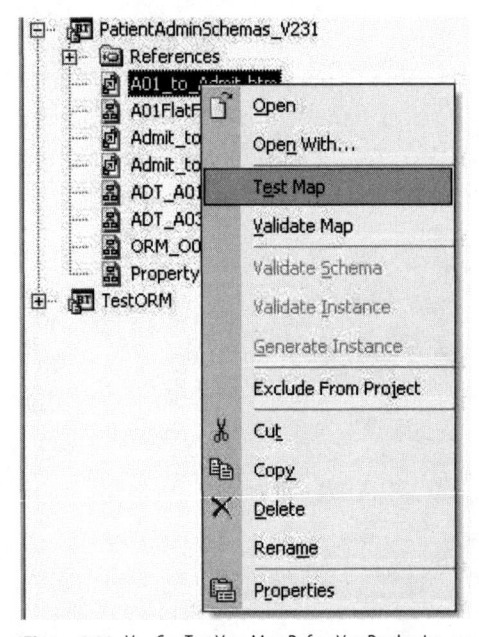

Figure 8.19: You Can Test Your Map Before You Deploy It.

3. Once you are satisfied with your map output, you are ready to deploy the map project. To do this, first add an assembly key file to the project, then right-click on the project and select **Build and Deploy**. Once deployed, the map can be called via a receive port, as part of an orchestration Transform shape, or via a send port.

> **NOTE**
>
> Because BizTalk relies on XML data for map processing, all maps called via a send port occur on the data before the ASM serialization. This is helpful to keep in mind when coordinating map outputs.

When using a map to create HL7 data, you will need to call that map through an orchestration in order to assign the **MSH** Segment to the data once it is transformed. To do this, you will need to add a Construct shape to an orchestration that calls the transformation map that creates the body of your message. After that, the data will flow to another Construct shape that assigns an **MSH** Segment to the beginning of the message. Figure 8.20 shows the data flow through an orchestration. The orchestration then sends the combined data to whichever send port(s) you specify. For complete details on this process, please refer to the Message Enrichment Tutorial contained in the BizTalk Accelerator for HL7 Help files.

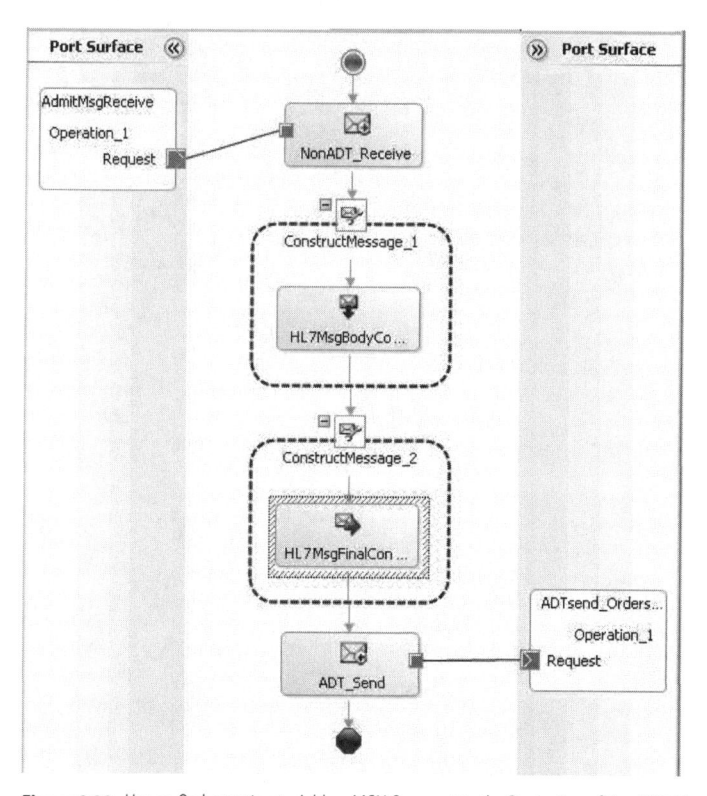

Figure 8.20: Use an Orchestration to Add an MSH Segment to the Beginning of Your HL7 Message.

Summary

This chapter has briefly described how the BizTalk Accelerator for HL7 addresses the unique business challenges raised by HL7 data processing. When working with the BizTalk Accelerator for HL7, it is important to remember that you are actually working with the entire BizTalk product, which means that you have all BizTalk features at your disposal. Together, they make for a robust solution to your integration challenges.

Chapter 9

Integration Challenges of HIPAA

The Health Insurance Portability and Accountability Act of 1996 (HIPAA) was the result of efforts by the Clinton Administration and congressional healthcare reform proponents to reform healthcare in a way that would streamline industry inefficiencies, reduce paperwork, make it easier to detect and prosecute fraud and abuse, and ensure greater privacy in our healthcare experience.

HIPAA affected healthcare EDI in the United States because one of its provisions required the Department of Health and Human Services (DHHS) to adopt national uniform standards for the electronic transmission of certain health information. In addition to the introduction of rigid data standards, HIPAA affected healthcare integration plans through the introduction of strict security and privacy requirements for the sharing and storage of healthcare data.

In 1996, when HIPAA was implemented, healthcare costs were rising at roughly twice the inflation rate. The high cost of healthcare was associated with administrative inefficiencies arising from the many entities that share information, because most of the information was shared in a manual form or through different electronic formats. All in all, administrative costs were estimated at about 20% of a typical healthcare bill.

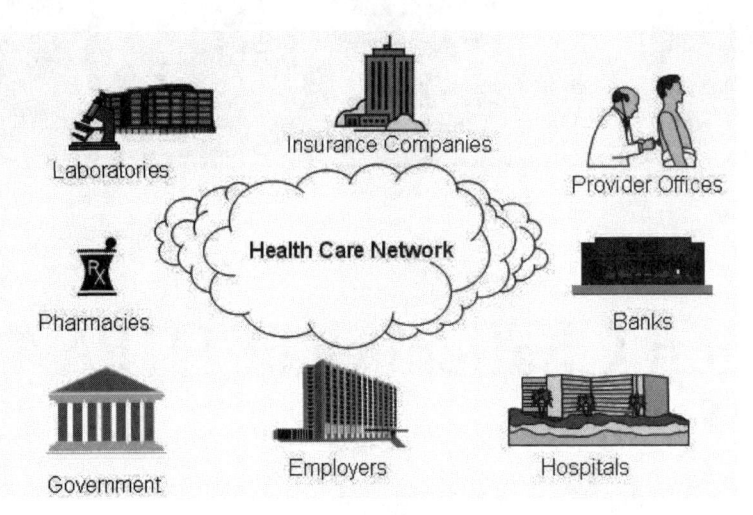

Figure 9.1: Typical Entities that Share Healthcare Information on a Daily Basis.

Additionally, as seen in Figure 9.1, many entities regularly share healthcare data. With so many parties handling healthcare data, the security and privacy of patient data was an issue that needed resolution. HIPAA provides many challenges for healthcare data integration because of the strict nature of its EDI regulations along with its stringent requirements to provide for the security and privacy of patient data.

A further challenge is that future EDI regulations under HIPAA require linking HL7-formatted data within the HIPAA-mandated structure for some documents. For many entities currently processing HIPAA data, this will necessitate incorporating a formerly distinct and foreign data structure into their daily integration processing.

Rules that Affect the Healthcare Industry in the United States

The rules that affect the healthcare industry in the United States come from the Administrative Simplification provisions under Title II of HIPAA. These provisions are aimed at reducing administrative costs and burdens in the healthcare industry by adopting and requiring the use of standardized, electronic transmission of administrative and financial data that was currently executed manually and on paper.

Administrative simplification is a method of making business practices (billing, claims, computer systems and communication) uniform, so that providers and payers do not have to modify the way in which they interact with each other through proprietary systems.

At the time HIPAA was implemented, it was estimated that over 400 different formats were used to accomplish six basic tasks:

- Enrolling an individual in a health plan
- Paying health insurance premiums
- Checking eligibility
- Obtaining authorization to refer a patient to a specialist
- Processing claims
- Notifying a provider about the payment of a claim

On average, 26 cents of every healthcare dollar was being spent on administrative overhead to accomplish these tasks.

Healthcare EDI

Computer-to-computer exchange of information in a standard format is called Electronic Data Interchange (EDI). HIPAA mandates the use of EDI as a method of achieving administrative simplification. It requires providers, insurers, payers, and to a small extent, employers, to submit enrollments, eligibility, and claims processing via EDI transactions.

EDI is essentially a set of very specific rules governing how information will be packaged in order to send business documents such as orders, invoices, statements and payments electronically from one company (or electronic trading partner) to another.

EDI has been in use commercially since the 1980s. Most companies in the retail and manufacturing industries use EDI to process orders, send invoices, and issue or receive payments with their electronic trading partners.

Properly done, EDI transactions minimize human intervention and should process very quickly.

The theory behind the administrative simplification provisions of HIPAA is that providers should be able to submit eligibility or benefit inquires and claims via EDI transactions to the payer, whose claims system should process the EDI transaction quickly, returning a claim payment/advice electronically without delay.

Prior to HIPAA, electronic data formats were widely used in the healthcare industry, but the variety of data formats caused many processing delays between entities.

HIPAA seeks to simplify and encourage the electronic transfer of information by replacing many of the current nationally used non-standard formats with a single set of electronic transactions that would be used throughout the healthcare industry.

Affected Healthcare Transactions

Standardized formats and data content are required for the following transactions:

- Premium payments
- Enrollment and disenrollment in a health plan
- Eligibility inquiry and response
- Referrals and authorizations
- Claims/encounter data
- Claim status inquiry and response
- Payment and remittance advice
- Coordination of benefits
- First report of injury
- Claim attachments

Standards for first report of injury and claim attachments have not been finalized as of this writing, but are expected shortly. When they are implemented, we will see the first real blending of the HIPAA and HL7 data standards, with the claim attachment accomplished by embedding an HL7 message in the HIPAA transaction set.

These standards apply to all health plans, healthcare providers who choose to do business electronically, and all clearinghouses.

Entities that pay healthcare claims, as well as the providers and clearinghouses exchanging electronic payment information with each other, are all affected by HIPAA's requirements.

Impact on the Healthcare Industry

The HIPAA requirements have already had a significant impact on all aspects of healthcare delivery. As the law and requirements mature, standardizing healthcare transactions will impact everyone who is involved in exchanging healthcare information.

The scope of the HIPAA legislation may require a total systems renovation for some entities depending on the age and architecture of the individual applications.

Technology has experienced tremendous growth, making EDI an essential tool for conducting business in today's market. Two factors have contributed to this: the Internet and standardization. The development of standards has increased EDI capability with Internet protocols. By engaging in EDI, healthcare partners can improve relationships with their current trading partners and increase electronic business with others who have been unable, or unwilling, to do business electronically in the past.

Affected Entities

Healthcare information flows between Providers, Health Plans and Sponsors. The HIPAA-regulated EDI standards apply to any of these entities that currently store or exchange data in an electronic format.

Providers

Providers include entities such as physicians, hospitals and other medical facilities or suppliers, dentists, and pharmacies, and entities providing medical information to meet regulatory requirements.

Under the Federal Register, "a provider means a provider of services as defined in section 1861(u) of the Social Security Act, a provider of medical or other health services as defined in section 1861(s) of the Social Security Act, and any other person who furnishes or bills and is paid for health care services or supplies in the normal course of business."

Health Plan

Health Plans refer to a third-party entity that pays claims or administers the insurance product or benefit.

Under the Federal Register, "a health plan means an individual or group plan that provides, or pays the cost of, medical care." For example, a health plan may be an insurance company, health maintenance organization (HMO), preferred provider organization (PPO), government agency (Medicare, Medicaid, Civilian Health and Medical Program of the Uniformed Services (CHAMPUS), etc.) or an entity such as a third-party administrator (TPA) or third-party organization (TPO) that may be contracted by one of those groups.

Sponsor

A sponsor is "the party or entity that ultimately pays for the coverage, benefit or product. A sponsor can be an employer, union, government agency, association, or insurance agency.

Figure 9.2 shows the typical transaction flow between healthcare entities.

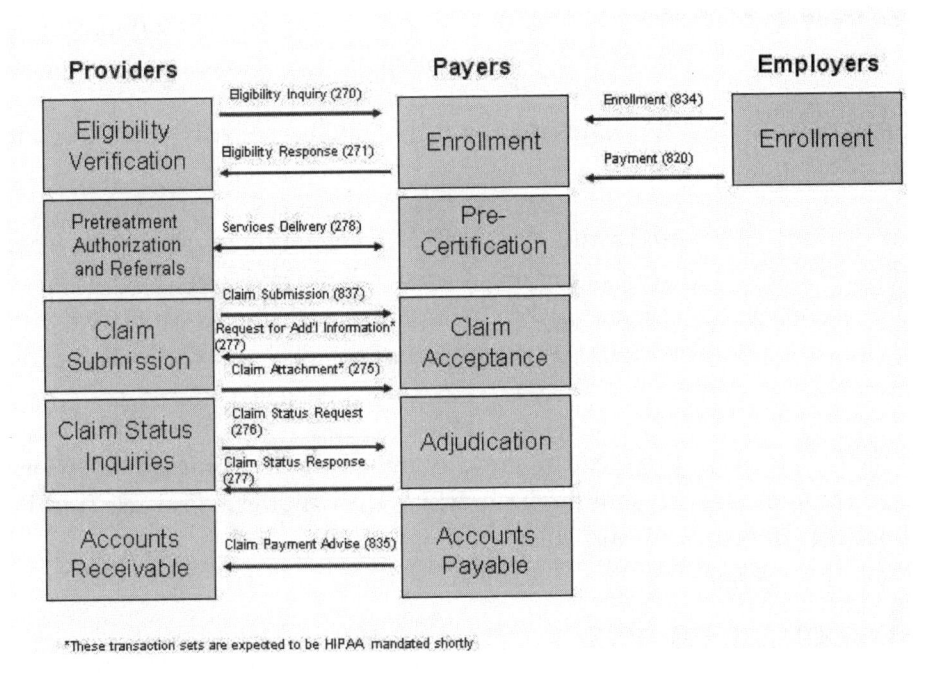

Figure 9.2: Transaction Flow Between Healthcare Entities.

Overview of HIPAA Standards

HIPAA addresses two aspects of data content standardization:

- Data elements, including their formats and definitions

- Standardization of the code sets or values that can appear in selected data elements:

  - ICD Diagnosis Codes

  - CPT Procedure Codes

  - HCPCS Procedure Codes

  - CDT Procedure Codes

  - NDC Drug Codes

  - Others

The standardization of data formats and definitions ensures that healthcare transactions can be shared between healthcare entities with minimal human intervention.

The standardization of code sets ensures that once the data is received by an entity, it will be processed accurately.

The American National Standards Institute's (ANSI) X12 standards, Version 4010, were chosen for all transactions except retail pharmacy transactions. However, the law allows for a different version of the X12 stadnard to be adopted annually. As of this writing, Version 4010 is the required version, but more recent versions form the basis for the revisions currently being evaluated.

Internet transactions are being treated the same as any other electronic transmission. However, there are some transmission modes in which the data format is irrelevant. In those situations, the data content must still conform to the standard.

Required Transaction Sets

The healthcare transactions mandated by HIPAA are numbered using a system that matches the non-healthcare EDI transaction identification scheme used with ANSI X12 data. They are often referred to simply by their numbers rather than their descriptive names.

The HIPAA mandated healthcare transactions are listed below with their associated numbers:

- 270 Eligibility Inquiry
- 271 Eligibility Response
- 275 Claim Attachment
- 276 Claim Status Request
- 277 Claim Status Response (Request for Additional Information)
- 278 Healthcare Services Delivery
- 820 Payment Order
- 834 Enrollment

- 835 Claim Payment
- 837 Claim

Introduction to the HIPAA Data Structure

The ANSI X12 standard (and thus the HIPAA standard) contains two main types of data: control data and the actual business data being exchanged, as shown in Figure 9.3. Control data is used to both route data and ensure accuracy as the data is being electronically transmitted. The business information being exchanged is the equivalent of documents traditionally used in business.

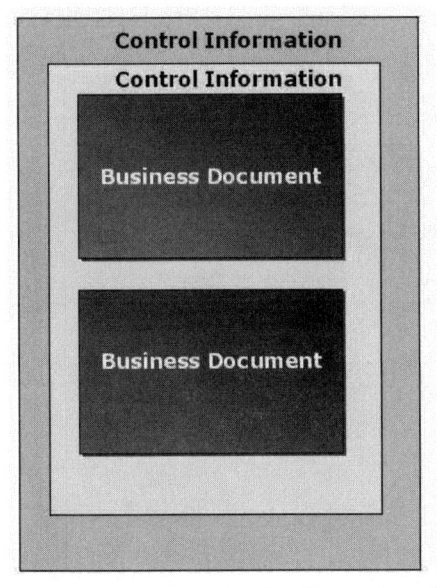

Figure 9.3: Some Data in the HIPAA Structure Serves Only as Control Information.

Data Components

Looking at Figure 9.4, you can see that HIPAA data can appear more complicated than it really is. To fully understand it, the data should be considered in pieces.

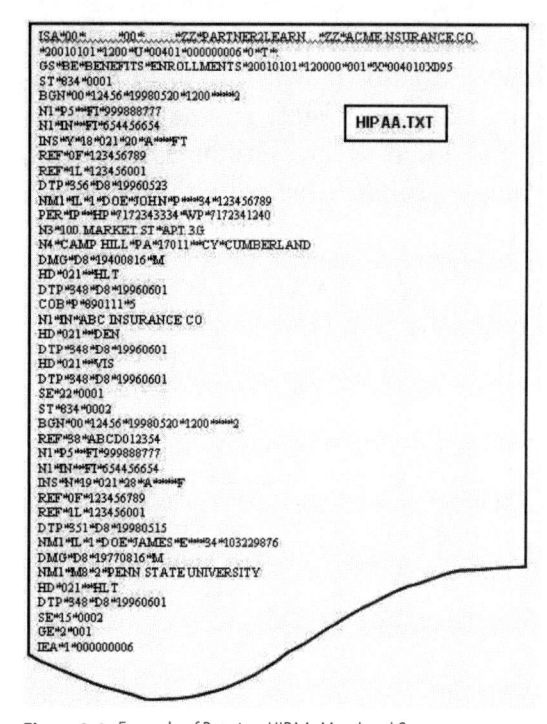

Figure 9.4: Example of Data in a HIPAA-Mandated Structure.

Elements

The smallest unit of data in the EDI structure is called an *element*. An element is the equivalent of a field. Some elements contain the same information as fields from an internal business application. However, a good number of elements are used as indicators of what the data in a subsequent element represents.

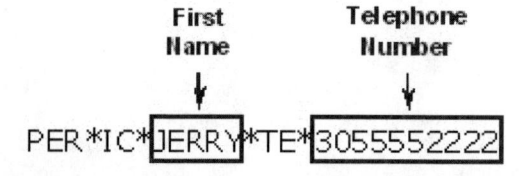

Figure 9.5: Data Elements.

To maximize file space, elements are often paired together, with one element serving as a qualifier to the other. The qualifier is limited to a specific set of values. The value of the qualifier then tells the reader what the data in the following element means.

For example, in Figure 9.5 above, the **TE** value in the third element indicates that the next element will be a telephone number. If you saw an **FX**, then the next element would be a facsimile number.

Every element used in ANSI data is named and has specific size and presentation requirements. However, they are typically referred to by their position in the segment. For example, the **First Name** element shown in Figure 9.5 is officially called **Name Element** but it is referred to as the PER 02, as it appears as the second element in the **PER** Segment.

Segments

Just as related fields are grouped into records in standard applications, related elements are grouped into segments in EDI. There are many different kinds of segments. Each kind of segment is identified by a Segment ID that appears at the beginning of the segment, as shown in Figure 9.6.

PER Segment

PER*IC*JERRY*TE*3055552222

Segment ID

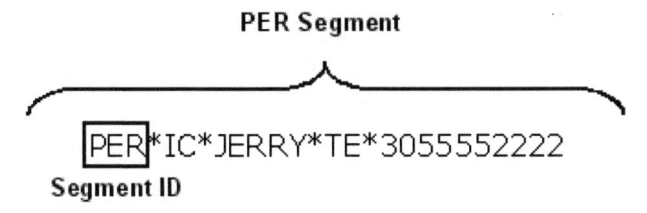

Figure 9.6: Data Segment.

Segments with the same Segment ID can appear in different places in the overall data structure. However, they represent different information depending on where they appear.

Transaction Sets

The business data exchanged between trading partners is included in a part of the EDI structure called a *transaction set*. The information included in a transaction set is the same as the information in a conventionally printed document. The transaction set is the actual business data being exchanged. As seen in Figure 9.7, many transaction sets will be present in a single EDI file.

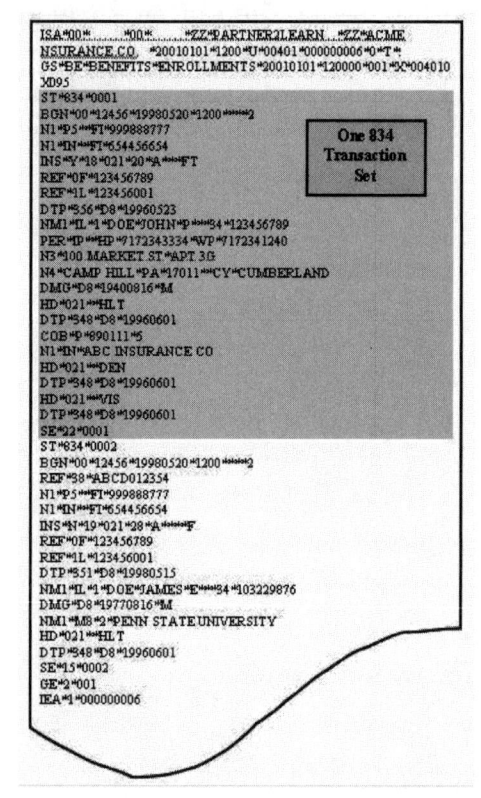

Figure 9.7: One EDI File Will Contain Many Transaction Sets.

Transaction Sets are identified by number. In EDI parlance, common business documents are referred to by their relative transaction set number. For example, a Claim is referred to as an "837," while an Eligibility Request/Response is referred to as a "270/271."

Each transaction set begins with an **ST** segment and ends with an **SE** segment.

The **ST** segment identifies the kind of transaction set because the transaction set number appears in the first element. For example, as seen in Figure 9.8, a healthcare claim would have "837" in the first element. The second, and last, element contains a sequential number identifying this transaction set specifically. The **SE** segment contains control information that ensures the integrity of the data.

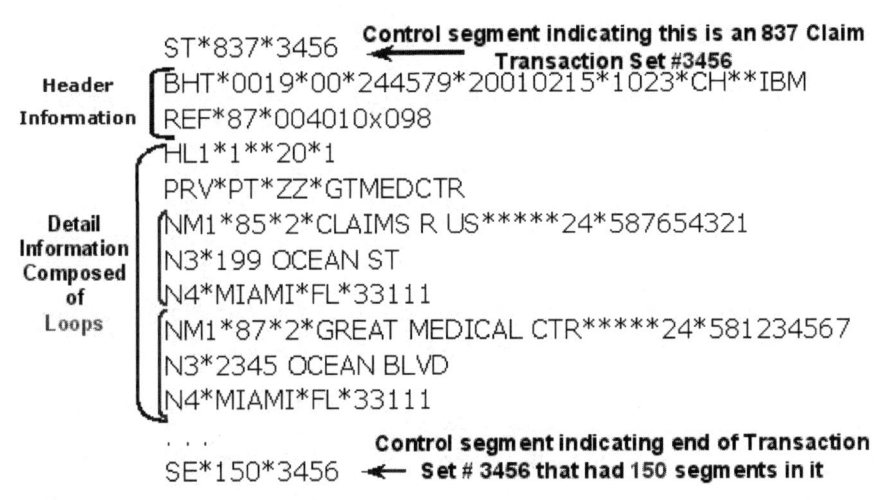

```
                    ST*837*3456         Control segment indicating this is an 837 Claim
                                        ←——— Transaction Set #3456
    Header         ┌BHT*0019*00*244579*20010215*1023*CH**IBM
   Information     └REF*87*004010x098
                   ┌HL1*1**20*1
                   │PRV*PT*ZZ*GTMEDCTR
     Detail        ┌NM1*85*2*CLAIMS R US*****24*587654321
  Information      │N3*199 OCEAN ST
   Composed        └N4*MIAMI*FL*33111
       of          ┌NM1*87*2*GREAT MEDICAL CTR*****24*581234567
      Loops        │N3*2345 OCEAN BLVD
                   └N4*MIAMI*FL*33111

                   . . .                Control segment indicating end of Transaction
                    SE*150*3456         ←——— Set # 3456 that had 150 segments in it
```
Figure 9.8: Transaction Set.

Transaction Set Details

Just as with any business document, each transaction set will have header, detail, and trailer information.

Segment Meaning

Each segment in the transaction set has a specific meaning. The reader can quickly determine the type of data contained in the segment by the segment ID. For example, a segment with a **PER** ID (called a *PER Segment*) will always contain contact information. A segment with a **DTM** ID (called a *DTM Segment*) will always contain date and time information.

Some segments need other segments to make them relevant. In this case, they are grouped together by an additional number in the Segment ID, as with the **NM1, NM2, NM3,** and **NM4** Segments. The **NM** segments always contain name and address information. The 1-4 numbers correspond to the different lines of an address.

Loops

Segments that are related in some way (where they need information from other segments to make them relevant) are grouped into objects called *loops*. A loop is simply a group of related segments. Sometimes the loop is identified by the segments it contains, as with the NM1 Loop.

Sometimes, the loop itself has a header segment to indicate its beginning. The **LX** Segment indicates a loop header.

Data Meaning

A segment's id indicates its specific purpose. Further, the data takes on additional relevance based on where it occurs in the data structure.

For example, an NM1 Loop always contains name and address information. However, if the NM1 Loop appears after a segment indicating the insured's information, it is the name and address of the insured. If the NM1 Loop appears after a segment indicating the provider of services information, it is the name and address of the provider.

Nested Loops

Healthcare data is complicated by the fact that there are usually three parties who need to be identified and tracked to ensure accuracy: the insured, the provider of services, and the insurance plan. Because of this, most healthcare transactions add meaning to their segments and loops by nesting them.

Nesting is essentially like outlining the data. Following a compositional hierarchy, details are related to the details they follow in the data stream.

For example, with claim information, the parent loop will be the provider who is making the claim. Inside of that, or following that in the data stream, is information on the insured's plan information. Following that is the information on the claim. Following that is a service line for each procedure being billed.

Through nesting loops, a few basic segments provide all the information needed to accurately detail a transaction.

Control Data

In addition to the business data being exchanged, files being sent electronically must specify:

- Who is sending the data and where it is going

- When the data was sent

- Once received, which internal department it should be routed to

Along with routing information, data must contain control indicators to ensure file integrity. Two structural levels are used to accomplish the data control needs:

- **Functional group** — in which related transactions appear

- **Interchange** — in which all the contact information for a single trading partner is placed

The Functional Group

Because trading partners may wish to exchange more than one kind of business document (such as instance claims and patient information) the *functional group* level was added.

All transaction sets of a specific type are bundled into a functional group. One functional group will contain all functionally related transaction sets. For example, all claims being sent are placed in a one functional group, while all eligibility requests being sent are placed in a second functional group.

A functional group begins with a **GS** segment. The first element in this segment indicates what kind of transaction sets are contained in this functional group. The rest of the information in the **GS** segment serves as internal routing instructions, tells the date and time of transmission, and identifies the version being followed.

The **GE** segment serves the same purpose as the **SE** segment—it indicates the end of the functional group, tells the number of included transaction sets, and has a control number that matches a control number in the **GS** to ensure data integrity.

A functional group is simply a group of functionally related transaction sets. For example, as in Figure 9.9 below, all 837's being transmitted by a provider will be grouped into one functional group. All 270's transmitted from this same provider would be in a separate functional group.

```
Tells what kind of documents follow and how they should be routed
   ──▶ GS*HC*001166999*3178884444*20010308*10
       5800*203*X*004010X098
      ┌ ST*837*3456
      │ SE*150*3456
      │ ...
      │ ...
      │ ST*837*3457
      └ SE*28*3457
   ──▶ GE*4*203
   Control segment indicating end of Functional Group # 203 that
                 contained 4 transaction sets
```

Figure 9.9: Functional Group.

The Interchange

Finally, an outside layer for data coming from a specific trading partner is called an *interchange*. All the electronic data being exchanged from a specific trading partner, or entity, is bundled into one interchange.

The first segments of both the interchange and any included functional groups are referred to as the "enveloping layer" because they serve the same purpose as envelopes do with conventional mail.

An interchange will have an enveloping layer that serves to route the data, and then it will have one or more kinds of business documents from this one trading partner. It begins with an **ISA** segment and ends with an **IEA** segment. There are three optional segments appearing in the interchange immediately after the **ISA** segment: the **ISB**, **ISE**, and **TA1** segments.

The **ISA** segment serves a similar purpose as that of an envelope to be mailed. It identifies where the data is going and who is sending it. Then, the three optional segments act similarly to any special mailing instructions you might place on your envelope. It contains information about:

- Who is sending the data
- Who the data should go to
- The date and time the data was sent
- What delimiters and terminator will appear in the data
- Whether this is test or production data

The **IEA** segment serves as a control indicating the end of this particular interchange. To ensure data integrity, the **IEA** segment contains:

- The number of functional groups in the data
- A control number that matches a number in the **ISA**

The **ISA** segment contains all the information about which business is sending this data, which business it is going to, the delimiters and terminator that will appear throughout the interchange, and specific formatting codes with information about the data.

The **IEA** indicates that this specific interchange is finished. It contains the same control number that appears in the **ISA** to ensure data integrity. In the raw data, every time you see an **ISA** segment you will know that the data to follow is from a new trading partner.

All Together

Overall, the EDI structure begins with control information and has the actual business data nested at the lowest level of the structure. The structure is similar to one business putting all the documents they want to exchange with a specific trading partner into a single box. That box is then specifically addressed so that it can reach the desired trading partner. For example, a box could say "To: ABC Co., From: XYZ Co."

Once the trading partner receives the box, it will find one or more envelopes inside. Each envelope is marked with the kind of business documents they contain and may have information about the internal department they should be routed to. For example, all the claims are in an envelope marked "Claims – Send to Adjudication."

When each specific envelope is opened, the business will find each individual business document. For example, when the Adjudication department opens its envelope, it will find a document containing five different claims.

In traditional EDI, the looping structure of certain transaction sets can get quite complicated. With healthcare EDI, the structure is further complicated by the fact that so many variables must be accounted for.

The specific requirements for the order of segments and whether they are optional or required are outlined in the HIPAA Implementation Guidelines, which are defined by the DPHS after considerable input from healthcare industry groups and published by the Washington Publishing Company (www.wpc-edi.com).

HIPAA's Other Rules that Affect Integration

There are several other HIPAA compliance rules currently defined and proposed but not yet finalized. These compliance rules involve standards designed to ensure the privacy and security of healthcare information.

Privacy Rules

The *Standards for Privacy of Individually Identifiable Health Information* are designed to help guarantee the privacy and confidentiality of patient medical records. The electronic transmission of medical information required by HIPAA has led to a general information revolution in the healthcare industry. While this revolution has led to many advances in patient care, it has also placed sensitive patient health information in the hands of more people than were ever involved with a paper-based system. The privacy standards adopted by HIPAA are designed around granting greater legal protection to an individual's right to privacy in health information than existed prior to the technological advancements brought on by the EDI requirements of the law.

The general concern was that the ease of information collection, retention, and exchange made possible by both modern day electronic technology and the EDI requirements of HIPAA would eliminate many of the logistical obstacles that previously served to protect the confidentiality of health information. The malicious interception of private health information for uses ranging from identity theft to prurient interest is much easier to accomplish when it is being exchanged electronically than when patient data was only available in paper form in a provider's office.

Even within a provider's facility, it was estimated that an average of 150 people ranging from medical to administrative staff had access to a patient's medical records during the course of a typical hospitalization. While many of these people have a legitimate need to view the patient's data, the drafters of HIPAA found it alarming that no laws governed who those people were, what information they were able to see, and what they were allowed to do with the information once they had access to it. The framers of HIPAA were aware of many instances of deliberate and accidental disclosure of individually identifiable health information, ranging from hospitals posting the medical records of thousands of patients on the internet to healthcare companies using patient data to solicit customers.

The privacy standards adopted by HIPAA are quite complex because they establish national minimum standards to protect the privacy of individually identifiable health information in prescribed settings. The standards address the varied uses and allowed disclosures of private health information by health plans, providers, and clearinghouses. The privacy standards have many provisions and are necessarily quite complicated when viewed on the whole, but when viewed in terms of the electronic exchange of data, they can be quite simply accommodated by HIPAA's accompanying security standards.

In terms of the electronic transmission of health data, the privacy standards delineate what type of information can be shared between entities. The accompanying proposed security standards enforce the privacy concerns because they limit how data is exchanged, which protects against unauthorized disclosure of information.

Security Rules

To supplement its privacy rules, HIPAA contains proposed technical and physical security rules designed to safeguard data integrity, confidentiality and availability. These security standards delineate the required steps to enforce:

- Access Control

- Audit Controls

- Authorization Control

- Data Authentication

- Entity Authentication

- Data Control

- Physical Equipment Access Controls

These security controls address both the physical location and protection of data along with use-based controls designed to ensure that information is viewed only by people with a legitimate need for access.

HIPAA's security rules fall into two categories: technical security provisions and physical safeguards. The physical safeguard provisions address such items as hardware access, data storage and backup plans, data disposal, and disaster recovery. However, the challenge in terms of a healthcare data integration strategy comes from the law's technical security provisions.

The technical security provisions address a variety of controls aimed at ensuring data access only by approved personnel, which in turn enforces HIPAA's privacy provisions. In terms of data access, the security standards require documented and enforced role-based and user-based access controls involving entity authentication during and after user access. Each entity must also put in place audit controls that record and examine system activity so that it can readily identify suspicious data access activities.

While context, user, and role based data access must be protected, the use of data encryption is optional. However, as technology advances and data is shared between entities via unsecured networks, encryption becomes a vital tool to enforce not only data access but also entity authentication—namely that a receiving or sending party is who it says it is.

A final security challenge in terms of data integration comes from proposed data authentication requirements. The data authentication provisions require that an organization be able to provide corroboration that data in its possession has not been altered or destroyed in an unauthorized manner. Entities can accomplish the required authentication level by including with the data a check sum, double keying, message authentication code, or digital signature.

Summary

HIPAA is a complex law with strict provisions. It certainly raises many challenges in terms of data integration, because the transaction and code requirements of its EDI provisions contain detailed mandatory data content and coding provisions. Furthermore, the security provisions meant to ensure data privacy challenge the integration architecture that is implemented, because it must allow for a variety of access and authentication controls. BizTalk Server 2004 is uniquely suited to meet these challenges because it links a robust integration tool with the security standards designed into the Microsoft .NET and Windows Server Platform.

Did you know?

The original wording of HIPAA allows for the Director of Health and Human Services to update the required electronic format of healthcare data every year. It is important to stay current with the latest HIPAA requirements.

A good source for current information on HIPAA is the Workgroup for Electronic Data Interchange, which can be found at `http://www.wedi.org`.

They maintain a directory of HIPAA resources that can be accessed directly at: `http://www.wedi.org/snip/public/articles/index%7E4.htm`.

Chapter 10

Using BizTalk Server 2004 for Your HIPAA Strategy

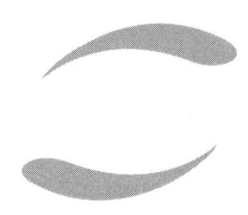

A HIPAA integration strategy involves much more than simply processing data in the mandated EDI format, referred to as the HIPAA Transaction and Code Sets (TCS). While this is a complex task in and of itself, the Microsoft BizTalk Accelerator for HIPAA 3.0 (HIPAA Accelerator) simplifies the process by providing a subsystem that allows BizTalk Server to receive a parsed HIPAA document structure represented as XML. Once formatted as XML, BizTalk can inspect the data, map the document into another form if necessary or initiate a business process in the form of a BizTalk orchestration. When leaving BizTalk Server, the Accelerator can once again be accessed to serialize the data into a HIPAA-formatted message. BizTalk enables the transmission of data between healthcare entities in a secure fashion.

Beyond basic TCS processing, BizTalk is the ideal solution as a HIPAA strategy because you have the ability to build security protocols directly into your TCS processing, rather than having to build those levels as pre/post processing steps. Through pipeline components that add encoding/decoding functionality, mandated security measures are integrated directly into your TCS integration, thus simplifying your overall HIPAA strategy.

Additionally, some HIPAA processing needs will involve transmitting or receiving non-HIPAA formatted data as supplemental information, commonly referred to as *supplemental files*. With BizTalk, there is no need to design a parallel architecture for supplemental files. BizTalk natively supports both flat file and XML-formatted file processing. Through orchestrations, supplemental files can be associated with or reconciled to their primary

HIPAA documents in a unified transaction, which eases auditing, logging, and troubleshooting activities.

Finally, as the HIPAA standard matures, we will likely see a blending of the need to process multiple data standards in a unified integration scenario. We are currently anticipating this development through the codification of new rules governing claims attachments. Claims attachments are meant to provide a HIPAA-mandated method for sending clinical documentation along with a healthcare claim. This clinical documentation will be in an HL7-prescribed format. Thus, in the near future, we will see a need to blend both HIPAA and HL7 processing. Given the flexibility provided by XSD schema definitions and BizTalk's inherent scalability as a publish/subscribe tool, it is an easy task to blend processing of diverse data formats for use with a variety of applications and trading partners.

This chapter provides an overview of the functionality of the HIPAA Accelerator in light of basic HIPAA transaction and code set processing. We will also look at how to build encryption/decryption security measures into your HIPAA processing. Armed with this HIPAA-specific information, along with the standard BizTalk information contained in Chapters 3 through 6, you will be able to design a thorough HIPAA integration strategy using BizTalk Server 2004.

The Microsoft BizTalk Accelerator for HIPAA 3.0

When processing HIPAA-mandated transaction and code sets, the first challenge to overcome is the receipt, validation, and acknowledgement of the data. When using BizTalk Server 2004, the next challenge is to parse the flat file formatted data into BizTalk's internal XML structure so that it is available for further processing by BizTalk components such as maps and orchestrations. Additionally, when using BizTalk to create HIPAA data, the data will need to be serialized into the HIPAA-mandated format for sending to your trading partners. This is where the Microsoft BizTalk Accelerator for HIPAA 3.0 (HIPAA Accelerator) comes in.

The HIPAA Accelerator is an add-on component to BizTalk Server 2004. The primary purpose of the accelerator is to enable the receipt, acknowledgement, and parsing of inbound HIPAA data as well as the serializing and transmission of outbound HIPAA data. The accelerator includes a HIPAA EDI subsystem that handles the document parsing and serializing of messages, as well as an adapter to connect to the subsystem. In addition, the HIPAA Accelerator provides the document specifications and components necessary to configure schemas for all of the HIPAA-mandated transaction sets. When you install the HIPAA Accelerator you will see a HIPAA EDI Adapter as well as HIPAA receive and send pipelines. Whether it is sent via the HIPAA EDI Adapter or a HIPAA pipeline, all data passes through the HIPAA EDI subsystem, where HIPAA data is validated according to HIPAA document definitions that are installed in the HIPAA EDI Repository.

In addition to the data validation and conversion that occurs in the HIPAA EDI subsystem, the HIPAA EDI Adapter enables the automatic and routine pickup of data from either a file or FTP location and routes the data to a specific receive location per sending entity. When sending data, the HIPAA EDI subsystem enables the creation of individual transaction sets that are then batched into an EDI format for transmission. When receiving or sending data via some other transport besides File or FTP (such as HTTP), you can still send data through the HIPAA EDI subsystem by routing the data through the HIPAA receive and send pipelines.

The HIPAA Accelerator also enhances the Health and Activity Tracking (HAT) database with a HIPAA EDI Reports view that provides auditing and logging information about all HIPAA data passed through the HIPAA EDI subsystem through either the HIPAA EDI Adapter or the HIPAA pipelines. This is enabled because all data passed through the HIPAA EDI Repository is stored in the BizTalkHIPAA_EDIDb database. Using the BizTalk HIPAA Administration Console, you can access properties for the HIPAA EDI Adapter which, among other things, allows you to configure automatic archival for the HIPAA data stored in the BizTalkHIPAA_EDIDb database.

Receiving Data Using the HIPAA EDI Adapter

To use the adapter provided by the HIPAA Accelerator you will choose the **HIPAA_EDI** transport type when configuring a receive location. Figure 10.1 shows a sample HIPAA EDI Adapter configuration on a receive location.

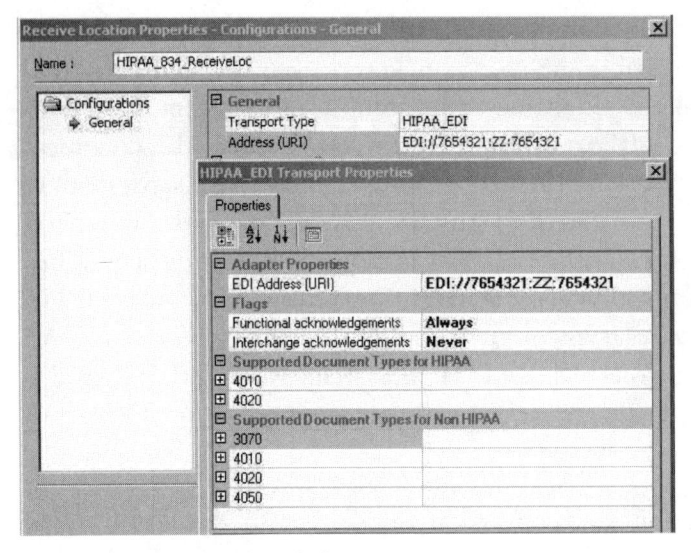

Figure 10.1: Sample HIPAA Adapter Configuration.

The HIPAA EDI Adapter uses BizTalk Party definitions to associate sending entity identifying values (found in the ISA Segment of the data) with a specific receive location for that sending entity. Thus, when processing HIPAA data, you will create a specific receive location for each entity (your trading partners) that you exchange data with. Figure 10.2 shows the receive locations that would be necessary if you receive HIPAA 837 professional claims from two trading partners, the Contoso and Northwind companies.

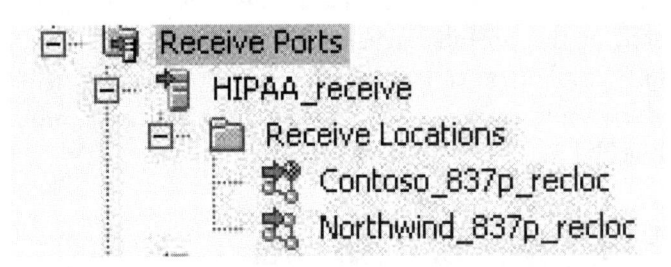

Figure 10.2: A Receive Location is Necessary for Each Trading Partner.

Follow these steps to configure the adapter:

1. If you are receiving data from both Contoso and Northwind, you will need to create two Party definitions in BizTalk Explorer (one for each company). Since you will need the Party definition in order to configure the receive location, you should create this first. To define a Party, right-click on **Party** in BizTalk Explorer and select **Add New Party**. A dialog box appears where you can name the Party entry. Configure the **Organization**, **Qualifier**, and **Alias** by simply typing the values into the appropriate column.

   In the **Party** definition, **Organization** and **Qualifier** are user-defined values that simply allow you to configure different EDI addresses for this particular Party. What is important is the **Alias** value. This value must always start with the `EDI://` moniker. The rest is composed of three parts, separated by a colon:

   - ISA value for the Party (this is mandatory)

   - ISA qualifier for the Party's identifier (optional)

   - Application id for the Party (found in the **GS** Segment and also optional)

   Figure 10.3 shows the Party definition for the Northwind Hospital whose ISA identifier is `1234567`, ISA qualifier is `ZZ`, and Application ID is also `1234567`.

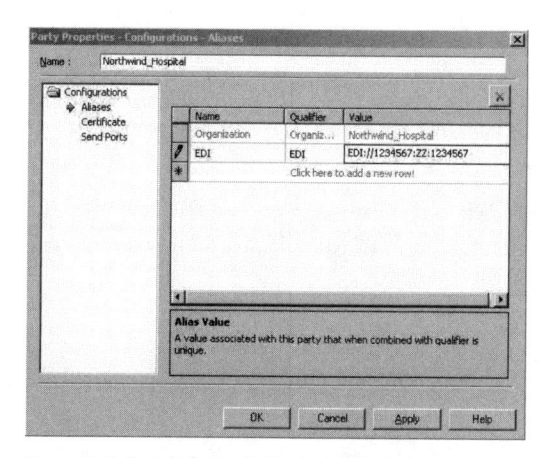

Figure 10.3: Party Definition for Northwind Hospital.

2. Once you have a Party definition for your trading partner, you can create a receive location for it. When creating the receive location, you will select **HIPAA_EDI** as the **Transport Type**, then click the browse button in the **Address (URI)** row. This will open up a dialog box, **HIPAA_EDI Transport Properties**, that you will use to configure the HIPAA EDI Adapter to accept HIPAA data coming from this particular trading partner (Northwind Hospital in our case).

3. In the **HIPAA_EDI Transport Properties** dialog box, use the browse button in the **EDI_Address** row to open a window displaying all of your Party definitions. You will select the Party definition for this trading partner. Figure 10.4 shows the Party choices available in our scenario.

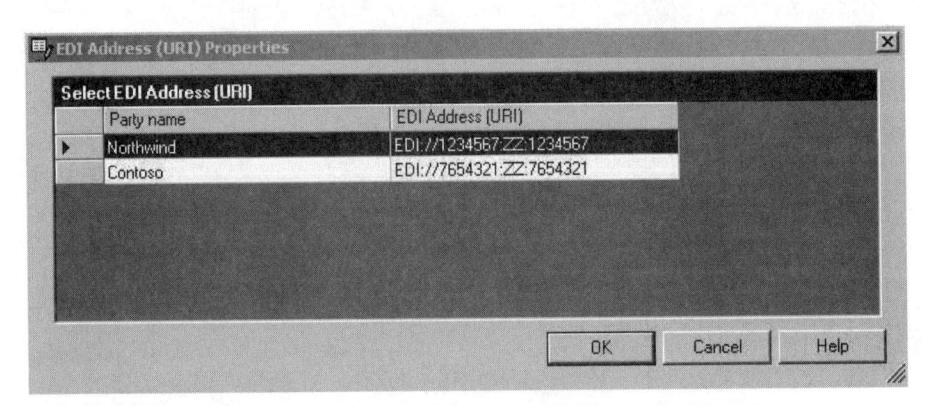

Figure 10.4: Party Definitions Available for Contoso and Northwind Receive Location Configurations.

4. Once you have selected the Party for whom you are configuring this receive location, you will return to the **HIPAA_EDI Transport Properties** dialog as seen in Figure 10.5 below. At this point you will configure the level of EDI acknowledgements that you wish to create based on data from this Party. Figure 10.5 depicts the configuration choice to create 997 Functional Acknowledgements to send for all data received from Northwind over this receive location.

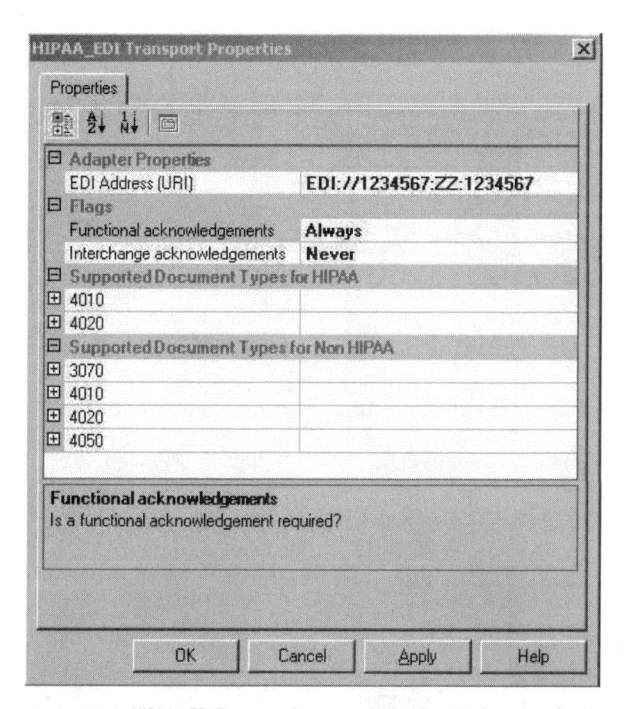

Figure 10.5: HIPAA_EDI Transport Properties Dialog Box Configuration for Always Creating 997 Functional Acknowledgements.

5. In the **Supported Documents** section, configure the type of documents that this party will be sending you. You can configure multiple documents at this time. To configure a document, select its row and then use the drop down arrow to select the enveloping structure that you expect to receive for these transaction sets. This secondary enveloping selection allows for data that may contain non-standard **ISA** Segments. Figure 10.6 below shows the selection of HIPAA 834 transaction sets that are expected to be wrapped in a version 4010-compliant **ISA** Segment.

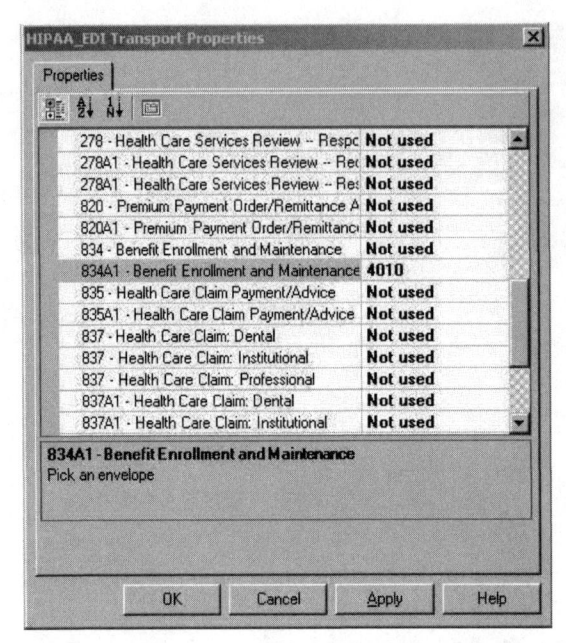

Figure 10.6: Configuration Enabling Receipt of HIPAA 834 Transaction Sets that Are Expected to Be Wrapped in a Version 4010-Compliant ISA Segment.

6. Once you have completed configuring the document types you expect to receive over this receive location, click the **OK** button to close this dialog box. To complete your receive location configuration, select the desired BizTalk Host Application and use the default **BizTalk PassThru Pipeline**. The reason to use this pipeline is because the HIPAA EDI Adapter sends the data through the HIPAA EDI subsystem, where the data is validated, so you do not need a pipeline for validation or serialization. Figure 10.7 shows your complete receive location configuration.

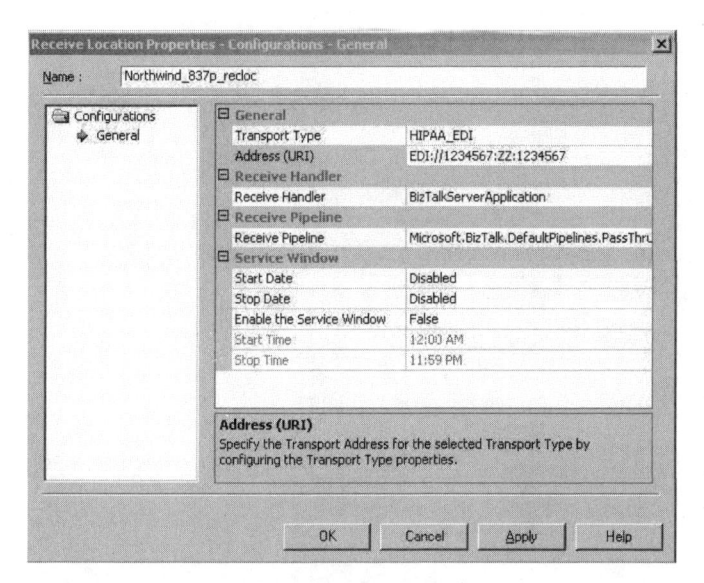

Figure 10.7: Completed Receive Location Configuration for the Northwind HIPAA Trading Partner.

Sending Data Using the HIPAA EDI Adapter

When using BizTalk to create HIPAA data, you will configure the HIPAA EDI Adapter on a send port in much the same fashion as when you configured it to receive data. Once again, you will select **HIPAA_EDI** as the **Transport Type** and access the **HIPAA_ EDI Transport Properties** dialog box by using the browse button in the **Address (URI)** row. As with receive locations, once the HIPAA_EDI Transport Properties are configured you will configure the send port as necessary, remembering to use the default **PassThruTransmit** pipeline. Figure 10.8 shows a send port configured to use the HIPAA EDI Adapter.

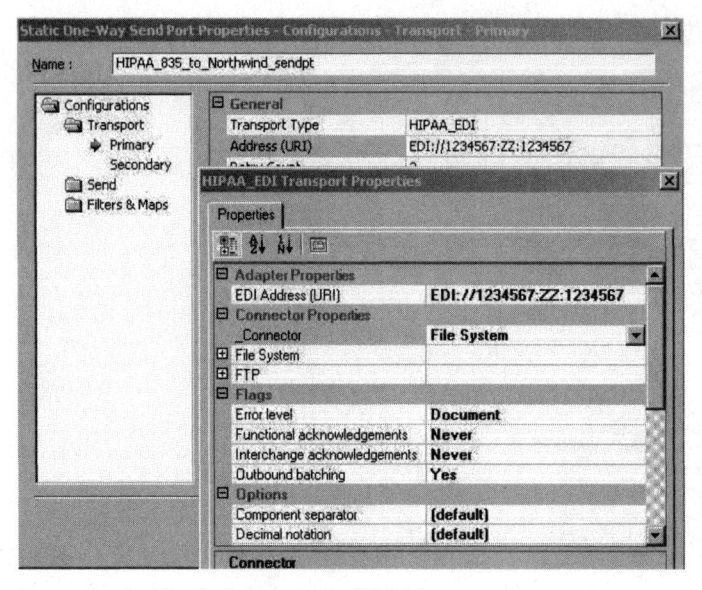

Figure 10.8: Send Port Configured to Use the HIPAA Adapter.

However, when sending HIPAA data, the HIPAA EDI Adapter requires more configuration than when receiving data because it will:

- Automatically send the data via FTP or to a file location

- Automatically batch HIPAA transaction sets into an EDI structure

- Use user-defined syntax values

- Wrap different transaction sets in different **ISA** Segments as desired

As seen in Figure 10.9, the **HIPAA_EDI Transport Properties** dialog box for a send port contains entries for configuration of each of these attributes.

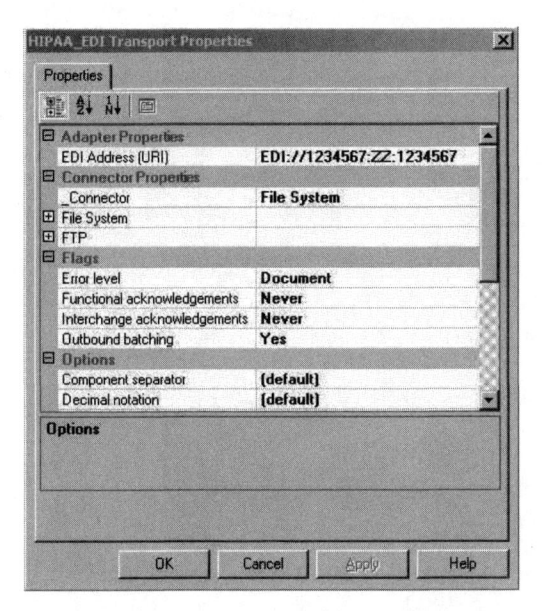

Figure 10.9: HIPAA_EDI Transport Properties Dialog Box for a Send Port.

Importing Document Definitions

The HIPAA EDI Adapter will receive HIPAA data and validate it against a document definition as EDI data. Next, the data will be converted into BizTalk's internal XML format before being passed into the BizTalk Messagebox. When sending data, a schema that defines the XML structure of the data will be used internally by BizTalk. Then, as the data passes through the HIPAA EDI Adapter, it is passed to the HIPAA EDI subsystem, where it will run through an internal map that will convert it from XML into its HIPAA flat file structure. The HIPAA Adapter refers to an EDI Repository to determine which document definition and internal map to use to validate and convert the data.

The next procedure in your HIPAA Accelerator configuration will be to import the document definitions expected to be received or sent into the EDI Repository. This will also import the mapping used to convert the XML document into an EDI representation. To import HIPAA document definitions, use the following steps.

1. Add an existing project to your Visual Studio .NET solution. Navigate to <installation drive>:\HIPAA install location\Microsoft BizTalk Accelerator for HIPAA 3.0\HIPAA_EDI\Adapter\EDI Schemas\004010A1and select the folder named for the transaction set you desire. From there, select the specific document definition for your data.

2. Once the schema opens in Visual Studio, you will import the document definition and associated EDI to XML mapping into the EDI Repository by validating the schema.

3. To validate the schema, right-click on it in the Solution Explorer and select **Validate Schema**. By validating the schema, you have successfully imported the schema into the EDI subsystem schema repository. At this point, your document definition and internal conversion map are installed into the EDI Repository for use by the HIPAA EDI Adapter.

Configuring System Settings for the HIPAA EDI Adapter

Your configuration to this point has involved setting up BizTalk to process specific data documents. You will now configure the HIPAA EDI Adapter to look in a specific directory for data that it will bring into a preconfigured receive location. Basically, you need to configure what's known as a *receive handler* for the adapter. The receive handler consists of file and FTP configurations known as *connectors*. The HIPAA EDI Adapter will poll these connectors every 30 seconds and send all documents found there into BizTalk.

Once the HIPAA EDI Adapter picks up data through a connector, it sends the data to the HIPAA EDI subsystem. The HIPAA EDI subsystem will:

- Validate the data according to the document specifications installed in the EDI Repository

- Determine the appropriate receive location to route the data to based on matching Party definitions to ISA identifiers

- Create EDI acknowledgments as necessary

- Run the data through a conversion map to create XML-formatted data for use by BizTalk internally

Chapter 10 - Using BizTalk Server 2004 for Your HIPAA Strategy

The HIPAA EDI Adapter then receives the document from the subsystem and sends it to BizTalk. Because of this, there is no need to use a special pipeline to route the data from the receive location to the message box. Rather, the data can simply be passed through "as is" to the message box after the HIPAA EDI subsystem processes it.

> **NOTE**
>
> This method works well when your data is received via a file drop or FTP. Should you receive data over HTTP or using SOAP, you will not use the HIPAA EDI Adapter. Rather, you will configure the HTTP or SOAP adapter as necessary and use the provided HIPAA receive pipeline to parse the data into BizTalk's internal XML format.

To configure the receive handler properties for the HIPAA EDI Adapter, use the following procedure:

1. From the **Start** menu, choose **Microsoft BizTalk Accelerator for HIPAA 3.0** ⇨ **BizTalk HIPAA EDI Administration Console**.

2. Under Microsoft BizTalk Server 2004\Adapters, select the HIPAA EDI adapter.

3. Under HIPAA EDI, select **Receive Handlers** and double-click the BizTalk host to open the **Properties** dialog.

4. Click the **Properties** tab and notice that the two entries under **Connector Properties** allow you to configure file and FTP pick-up information, as shown in Figure 10.10.

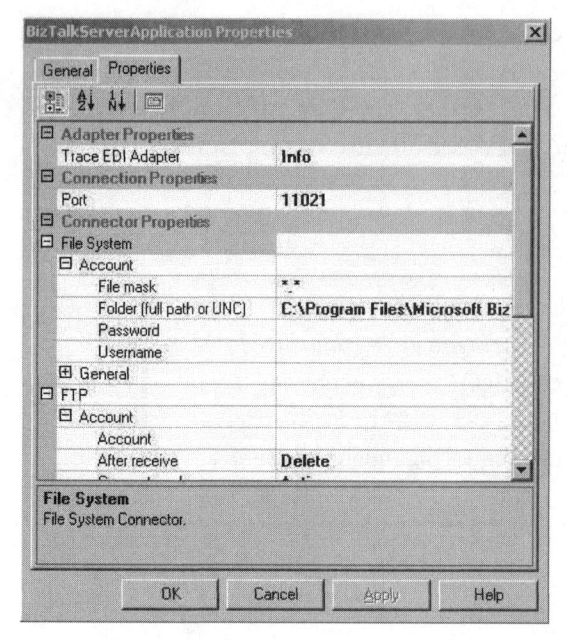

Figure 10.10: HIPAA EDI Adapter Receive Handler Properties Dialog Box.

The HIPAA EDI Adapter uses the connector information configured for the receive handler to locate data to send into BizTalk. Basically, the adapter polls these sites every 30 seconds. When it finds data, it picks it up and reads the **ISA** and **GS** segments to determine the sending party's information and the document type. It then searches through your receive locations for matching sending party and document information. The data is then run through the adapter's internal validation and conversion map and is sent into BizTalk as XML-formatted data. If the receive location has acknowledgements configured, then they are created at this time as well.

While the HIPAA EDI Adapter uses the receive handler properties to locate incoming data, it uses the send handler properties to identify the receiving party (your company's) identifiers. Also, when using BizTalk to create HIPAA data, the adapter will use the send handler configuration information to populate your company's ISA and GS information. You access the send handler properties by double-clicking on the BizTalk host for the send handler in the same fashion as with the receive handler's properties. Figure 10.11 shows the send handler configuration for your company's information, where your company is **ClaimsRUs** and has an ISA qualifier of **ZZ**, and ISA and GS values of **CLAIMSRUS**. Notice that to have your company's information available, you will also need to add a BizTalk Party definition for your company.

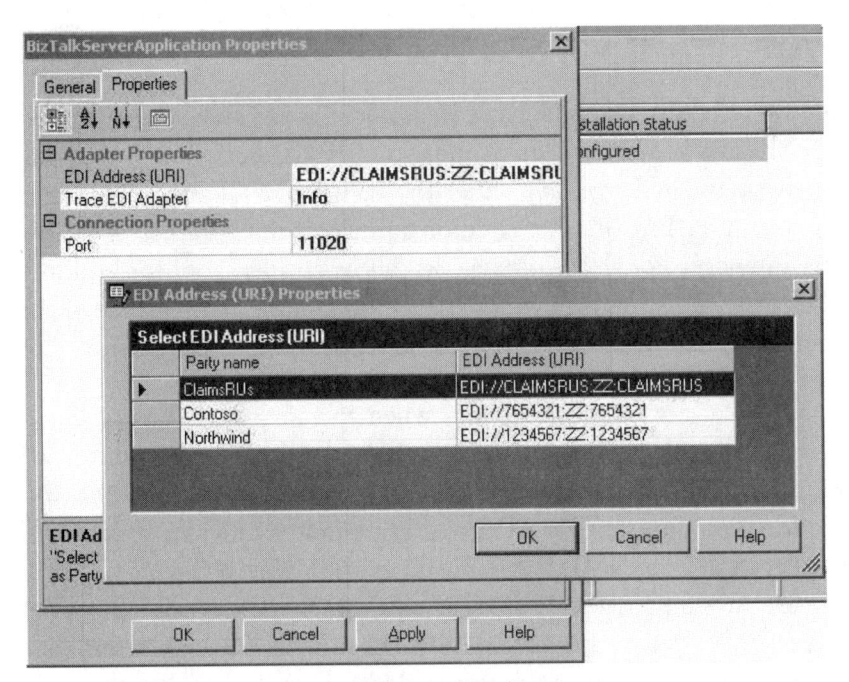

Figure 10.11: HIPAA EDI Adapter Send Handler Properties Dialog Box.

Because these configurations are used by the HIPAA EDI Adapter to locate data to send into BizTalk, validate sending and receiving party identifiers, and populate your sending party identifiers into outbound data, the HIPAA EDI Adapter receive and send handler properties will only need to be configured when you begin using the adapter or when your connection or EDI identifying information changes.

The HIPAA Accelerator documentation contains a complete tutorial on how to configure the HIPAA EDI Adapter to receive and send HIPAA-formatted data. The HIPAA EDI Adapter is convenient when you are using BizTalk to basically receive, route and send HIPAA-formatted data. However, because you use the BizTalk Pass Thru pipeline when using the HIPAA EDI Adapter, you will have a limited ability to map or perform business processing steps on the data. The next section discusses configuration steps for using the HIPAA pipelines instead of the HIPAA EDI Adapter.

Building HIPAA-Proscribed Security Measures

So far in this chapter, we have discussed the basic steps necessary to receive and process HIPAA data through BizTalk. However, there is more to HIPAA than simply receiving and routing data in the mandated format. Under the security requirements brought about by the privacy rules, a HIPAA implementation strategy is not complete if it does not include measures to encrypt or decrypt data. BizTalk is an ideal tool for building HIPAA's proscribed security measures into your HIPAA integration plan because of the ease in which you can add encryption/decryption information into your pipelines.

Essentially, you will need to create a custom pipeline when you are processing encrypted HIPAA data. Because of this, you will not use the HIPAA EDI Adapter as discussed earlier in this chapter. By using the provided HIPAA receive and send pipelines, you can receive the same functionality that the HIPAA EDI Adapter provides in terms of converting HIPAA data to and from XML. These pipelines are deployed when you install the HIPAA Accelerator and contain the HIPAA Disassembler (in a receive pipeline) and HIPAA Assembler (in a send pipeline) components. The HIPAA Disassembler/Assembler components send the data through the HIPAA EDI subsystem in the same way that the HIPAA EDI Adapter does. When using these pipelines instead of the HIPAA EDI Adapter, you are free to use whatever transport properties you desire, such as FILE, FTP, HTTP, or SOAP. You would then configure those transport properties as necessary. The data conversion occurs as the data runs through the HIPAA pipeline.

> **NOTE**
>
> The default HIPAA receive and send pipelines contain only the HIPAA Disassembler/Assembler components. You will use these pipelines instead of the HIPAA EDI Adapter when you need to run the data through a BizTalk map or orchestration.

> **FREE BONUS**
>
> A Payer Use Case for processing a HIPAA 834 transaction is available as a free download when you register this book at www.agilitypress.com.

When receiving encrypted HIPAA data, you will create a pipeline that is customized with the HIPAA Disassembler component as well as an encryption/decryption pipeline component. You will then use this customized HIPAA pipeline in the receive location that receives the encrypted HIPAA data.

To start the process, you will want to configure your system with the certificate information that will be used to validate the public and private key information that is encrypted on the data.

1. Configure your BizTalk Host with the certificate information by right-clicking it in the BizTalk HIPAA EDI Administration Console and selecting **Properties**. From there, configure the **Certificate** properties as desired. The **Thumbprint** property setting specifies which certificate, or private key to use when decrypting inbound messages (see Figure 10.12).

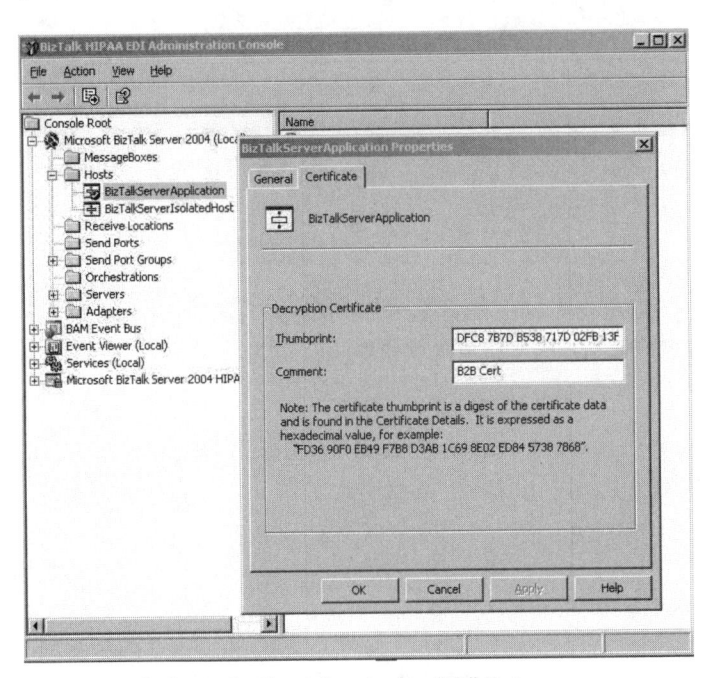

Figure 10.12: Configuring Certificate Information for a BizTalk Host.

2. Right-click on BizTalk Server (local) to associate a signing certificate with a BizTalk group. The **Thumbprint** setting here specifies which certificate to use when signing outbound messages. Once configured, you need to restart the BizTalk Server for the changes to take affect (see Figure 10.13).

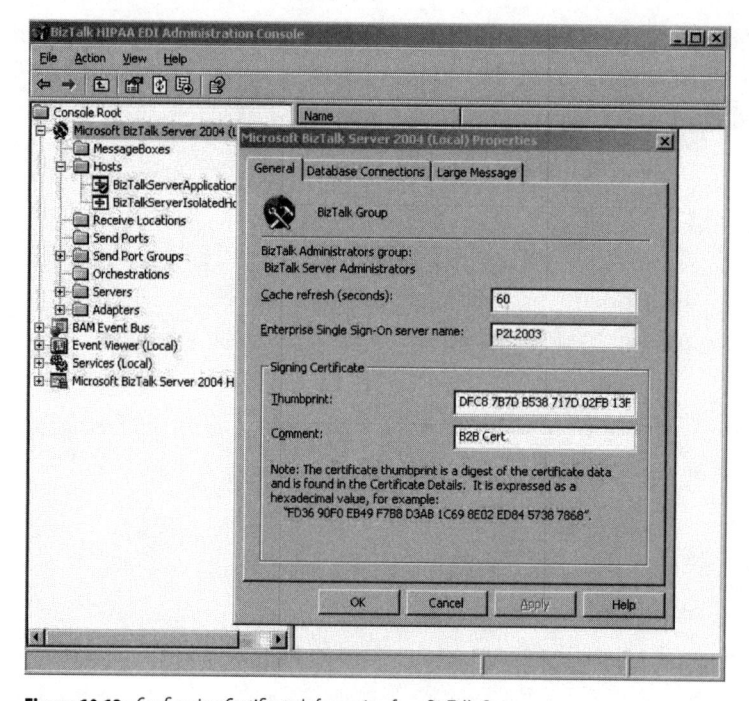

Figure 10.13: Configuring Certificate Information for a BizTalk Group.

The HIPAA Disassembler component performs data validation based on the document definitions in the EDI Repository and converts the data into BizTalk's internal XML format. This means that to process encrypted HIPAA data, you will need to add both the HIPAA Disassembler component and the MIME/SMIME Decoder component to a receive pipeline, according to the following steps.

1. Open a project to hold your custom HIPAA receive pipeline. Add a receive pipeline into the project as a **New Item**.

2. Once the pipeline opens, add the HIPAA Disassembler component by dragging it from the toolbox to the Disassemble stage of the pipeline.

3. Add the MIME/SMIME Decoder component to the pipeline by dragging it from the toolbox to the Decode stage of the pipeline. To configure it, right-click on the MIME/SMIME Decoder component, select **Properties**, and configure the necessary information as shown in Figure 10.14, such as:

   - Allow non MIME Message
   - Check revocation list

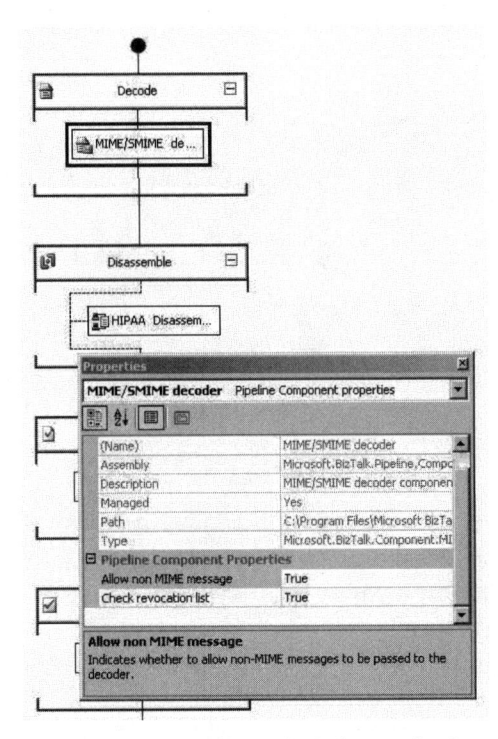

Figure 10.14: MIME/SMIME Decoder Configuration for a Custom HIPAA Receive Pipeline.

4. Once the MIME/SMIME Decoder component is configured, you will add the necessary assembly key file to the pipeline project and build and deploy it.

5. Create a receive location for the trading partner that you are receiving the encrypted data from. Use your newly deployed custom HIPAA receive pipeline for the pipeline choice in the receive location, as shown in Figure 10.15. As the data runs through the pipeline, it will be decrypted, validated, and converted before being placed in the BizTalk message database.

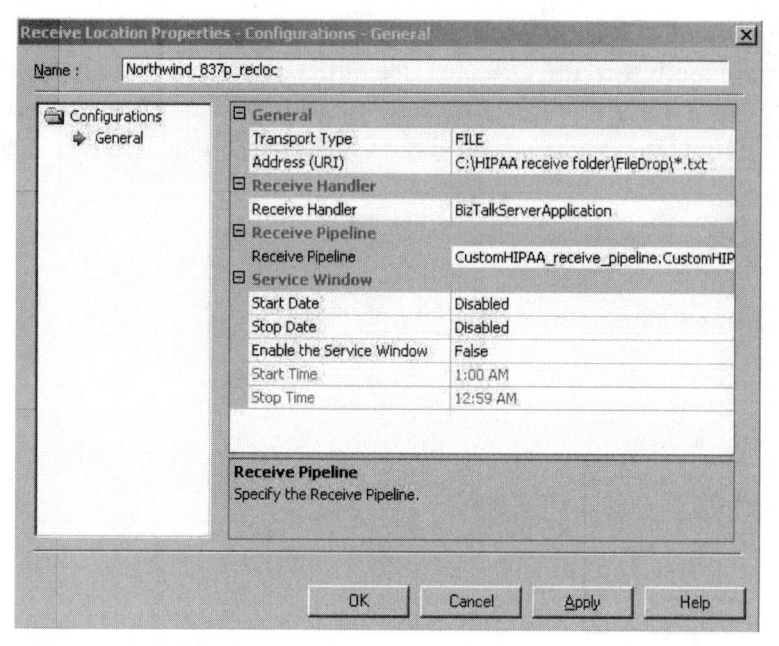

Figure 10.15: Receive Location Using a Customized HIPAA Receive Pipeline.

In order to send encrypted HIPAA data, you will need to customize a HIPAA send pipeline, according to the following steps.

1. Add a send pipeline to a new project. As with the custom receive pipeline, you will create a custom HIPAA send pipeline by dragging the HIPAA Assembler component into the Assemble stage of the pipeline.

2. Drag the MIME/SMIME encoder component from the toolbox into the Encode stage of the pipeline.

3. Right-click on the MIME/SMIME encoder component, select **Properties** and configure the necessary information as shown in Figure 10.16, such as:

    - Check Revocation List
    - Content transfer encoding
    - Enable encryption
    - Encryption algorithm

- Send body part as attachment

- Signature type

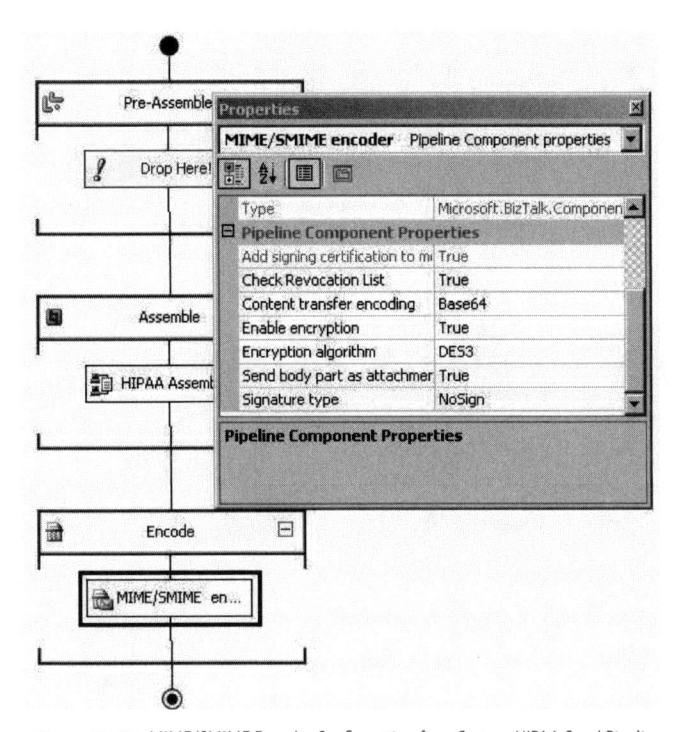

Figure 10.16: MIME/SMIME Encoder Configuration for a Custom HIPAA Send Pipeline.

As with a custom HIPAA receive pipeline, once the MIME/SMIME encoder component is configured, you will add the necessary assembly key file to the pipeline project and build and deploy it. Next, create a send port for use in sending the encrypted data. In that send port, use your newly deployed custom HIPAA send pipeline, as shown in Figure 10.17. As the data runs through the pipeline, it will be converted from XML to its proper HIPAA format, then encrypted before being placed in the send port transport location.

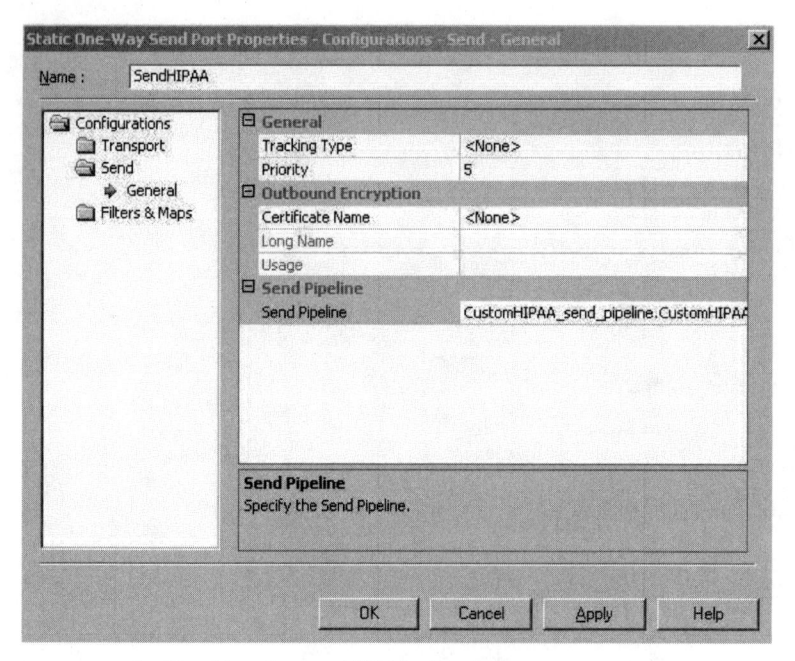

Figure 10.17: Send Port Using a Customized HIPAA Send Pipeline.

As you can see, when processing HIPAA data, you have a choice as to whether to use the HIPAA EDI Adapter or use a standard adapter but route your data through a HIPAA pipeline. Overall, the HIPAA EDI adapter provides greater functionality than the HIPAA pipeline, so it will likely be your preferred configuration choice. When using the HIPAA EDI Adapter, you will always use the default BizTalk PassThru pipeline. However, there will be instances where you will need to accept or send encrypted data. In these circumstances, it is nice to have the option to customize a HIPAA receive or send pipeline for your security needs.

Summary

As discussed in the introduction to this chapter, a complete HIPAA integration strategy involves more than the ability to receive and send HIPAA-formatted data. However, while not constituting a complete strategy, no HIPAA integration strategy can exist without this ability. BizTalk Server 2004, along with the Microsoft BizTalk Accelerator for HIPAA 3.0, provides the means to receive and send HIPAA data correctly. Beyond that, it enables you to have access to the complete functionality provided by BizTalk Server 2004 for designing additional solution needs, such as transformation maps, orchestrations, and even business activity monitoring. Together, BizTalk Server 2004 and the Microsoft BizTalk Accelerator for HIPAA 3.0 enable thorough HIPAA processing that not only complies with current TCS and security mandates, but provides a solution framework that will scale for future HIPAA processing needs.

Did you know?

You can configure properties for the HIPAA EDI Subsystem through the HIPAA EDI Administration Console.

In the HIPAA EDI Administration Console, select Microsoft BizTalk Server 2004 HIPAA EDI Adapter/Parameters at the bottom of the left navigation panel.

On the right side of the screen, select the HIPAA database on your BizTalk Server (it defaults to BizTalk HIPAAEDIDb).

Right-click on this database and select Properties.

You will see a series of tabs allowing you to configure many aspects of the HIPAA EDI subsystem, such as connector polling cycles, internal document numbering, and trace information.

Part III

Extras

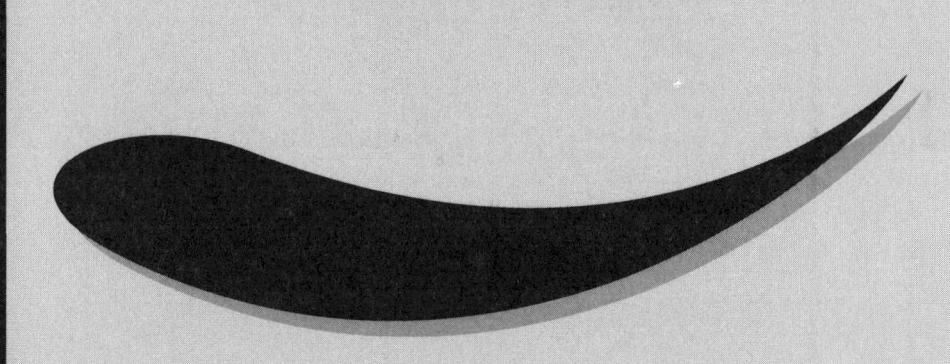

Appendix A

Fundamentals of Good Design

The ability to deploy multiple integration projects while keeping the overall architecture manageable requires a mix of flexibility and discipline. Maintaining the tenuous balance between making the overall architecture flexible enough to apply right technology to the requirements, and enforcing the discipline necessary for architectural consistency is one of the greatest challenges facing IT departments today. This chapter will outline several points that can help your organization successfully perform the high-wire act required of IT while enabling a platform for future growth.

Have an Integration Strategy

You can't design unless you have a clear idea what the end game looks like. To effectively manage a medium to large IT portfolio, you need a well-defined set of best practices along with a clearly articulated vision of how the architecture will grow and mature over time.

This vision of what you want your architecture to be allows you to focus on where to compromise and where to stand firm. Chapter 2 outlines several techniques for building an integration strategy.

Migrate Away From File-Based Integration

It is a best practice to migrate away from file-based integration to a messaging or service-based approach. Messaging technology has a very simple goal: to move data. Anytime you move bits around on your network (or even between applications on the same hardware), some sort of messaging is involved. However, all messaging techniques are not created equal.

While file transfer protocol (FTP) and files make up the majority of messaging used for interfaces today, they have some serious limitations, and should be used as a last resort. There are two main reasons why file-based messaging is not the best approach:

- **Loss of transactionality** — Any time one application relies on an outside application to do something, that's a transaction. When you use a file-based approach to integrate applications, there is no built-in concept of a transaction. As a result, you never know for certain if everything is synched up correctly. There is also no built-in way to control the order in which files are loaded. If you place an order and then update it, what happens if the update is loaded first? The current data is overlaid by the old data, resulting in an out-of-sync system. Even worse, you wouldn't know about it since neither application has a way to ensure that the transaction was executed in the right order.

- **Loss of data** — A second reason to avoid file-based integration is that you run the risk of losing data. What if the file is accidentally deleted?

A messaging layer provides you with the ability to move data around in a reliable, near real-time way. More specifically, a properly implemented messaging layer will do five things:

- Guarantee delivery of messages

- Give you a way to control the order in which messages are received (first in first out, last in first out, etc.)

- Give you some options on how messages are delivered, such as publish/subscribe, request/reply, broadcast, or point-to-point

- Allow the pieces of your infrastructure to communicate with each other in situations that have a high number of transactions

- Enable more advanced relationships between parts, such as two-phase commits and complex error handling

Often, organizations will have more than one messaging layer in use. While it is a good idea to consolidate these multiple messaging products into one, this approach is not always feasible. Recognizing this situation, BizTalk provides you with a number of options for implementing an enterprise-wide messaging infrastructure.

- Microsoft Message Queuing (MSMQ) is bundled as part of Windows, and provides an enterprise-class messaging layer. A MSMQ adapter is planned for BizTalk, and will provide off-the-shelf connectivity to MSMQ. In the interim, custom code can be inserted into the BizTalk transaction to provide this functionality. The advantage of using MSMQ is that it is already deployed on your Windows-based servers, and can be used across a wide variety of applications, resulting in architectural consistency.

- BizTalk Server 2004 ships with its own messaging layer, called BizTalk Message Queuing (MSMQT). MSMQT is essentially the same as MSMQ, except instead of sending messages to a queue, you send them to a BizTalk receive location. It is also important to note that MSMQT can send or receive messages to either local or remote private queues, but does not support public queues. The advantage of using MSMQT is simpler integration to the messaging layer for BizTalk-driven interfaces and the ability to handle message sizes over 4 MB.

- BizTalk Message Queuing-MQSeries Bridge provides connectivity to MQSeries in a similar fashion to the MSMQ-MQSeries Bridge. This bridge is useful when working with systems that do not have MSMQ or MSMQT available, such as a legacy system running a non-Windows operating system.

Use Smaller Transactions to Enable Better Business Visibility

It is a best practice to remove batched interfaces where possible and use smaller transactions to enable better business visibility. Since batched interfaces are viewed as one logical transaction, they are viewed by other layers of the architecture as one undifferentiated blob. As a result, you do not have the same visibility for BAM and orchestrations as you would if those transactions were processed separately.

Use Abstraction

It is a best practice to use abstraction and not access data sources directly. Abstraction is the process by which the physical aspects of a piece of data, message, or protocol are separated from the logical aspects. For example, an HL7 ADT^A01 message transmitted over MLLP are physical aspects of the logical event of a patient being admitted to a hospital. As you can imagine, if your components interact with the logical event instead of the physical aspects, they will be able to be reused, regardless of the format or protocol. In other words, the more components act upon abstract events, the more flexible the final solution will be.

Abstraction is the cornerstone of sustainable solutions. Abstraction allows for components to be reused, insulates business logic from system changes, and can significantly reduce the impact of changes on your system. From the standpoint of an integration architecture, there are three types of abstraction:

- **Abstraction at the protocol layer** — This is the most basic function of an integration platform. BizTalk provides a wide variety of adapters for receiving and sending messages, such as HTTP, MSMQ, and FTP. Protocol adapters allow you to easily work with messages coming from virtually any kind of transmission channel.

- **Abstraction at the data layer** — The mapping feature of BizTalk provides abstraction at the data layer. One way to do this is to use a common format for all messages that represent a business event or entity, otherwise known as a *canonical form*. A canonical form is an intermediate data structure which all data is marshaled to and from, as shown in Figure A.1.

The advantage of this approach is that it provides abstraction from the schema of the inbound message. Use BizTalk maps to help abstract various formats from the integration logic you use to route and process data.

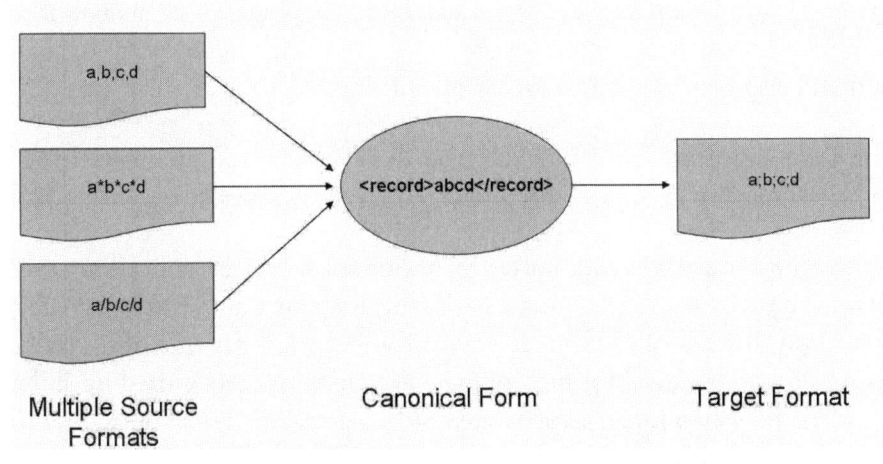

Figure A.1: A Canonical Form Can Be Used to Abstract the Formats of Inbound Messages from Target Systems.

- **Abstraction at the application layer** — This can be accomplished through the use of existing application program interfaces (API) that are part of a line of business applications. For those applications that do not have an API, try to avoid going straight to the database and directly issuing SQL statements. In these cases, build a web service to wrap database calls and expose the functionality required at a business level. This allows you to make changes to the underlying database schema without having to change any applications or interfaces that interact with the system.

Use Orchestration

Orchestration can be a powerful way to solve specific integration scenarios. If you have worked with previous versions of BizTalk, be sure to take another look at BizTalk orchestration. A lot of improvement has been made in this area of the platform, and you will be missing out on some very rich functionality if you neglect orchestration. See Chapter 5 for more information on orchestration.

Structure Projects to Have Multiple, Short Iterations

Regardless of the methodology you use to implement your projects, look for ways to break integration deliverables into small pieces that take less than four weeks to complete. Not only will this allow you to show the value of your work to the business sooner, it will also help you to manage project risk.

While necessary in just about any software deployment, requirements specifications tend to be less reliable in integration projects than other types of deployments.

Integration projects are typically started in response to a large application deployment. Too often, the focus for requirements gathering is spent on features and functions of the application, instead of looking at how the application fits into an overall business process. As a result, the need for integration sometimes isn't recognized until the project is well underway. When integration-related tasks are specified, few business analysts are skilled in understanding how to properly scope these requirements.

You can manage this situation through a project structured with many short iterations. The delivery of many small parts of a project instead of just one big delivery has the following benefits:

- Allows for timelier user feedback. Business users are more involved in the project because they will have more opportunities to provide feedback.

- Reduces project risk from so many moving parts and establishes a baseline of functionality.

- Encourages incessant testing of the end-to-end system, resulting in a more robust solution.

- Enables you to leverage the best practices of some of the leading experts of software project management through the use of agile software development methods.

Apply Agile Software Development Techniques

Because so many different systems are involved on most integration projects, change is constant. Interfaces change, application program interfaces change, and processes change. To be successful, you need to get your code into production quickly, and be able to rapidly roll out any changes to keep pace with the business. Waterfall methodologies (where all design must be complete before coding, and all coding must be complete before testing) often run into trouble when applied to integration projects because they do not account for the rapid rate of change. Waterfall approaches are good for highly structured projects with large teams and well-defined success criteria. Unfortunately, integration projects rarely meet any of these criteria.

On the other hand, agile software development techniques are ideal for integration projects because they encourage rapid rollout of smaller groups of functionality. A series of books has been written on the subject by Kent Beck that does an excellent job of covering how to apply agile software development to real-world projects. Refer to the "Further Resources" section at the end of this book for more information on this topic.

Appendix B

HL7 Version 3 Processing with BizTalk Server 2004

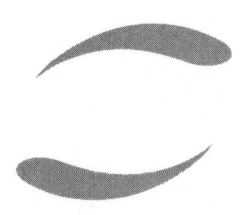

The BizTalk Accelerator for HL7 (HL7 Accelerator) was created specifically to process HL7 data formatted as Version 2.x data. As discussed in Chapter 8, the components provided by the HL7 Accelerator are required in order to meet the industry requirements for HL7 V2.x processing. Despite the fact that widespread adoption of HL7 Version 3 (HL7 V3) is still far off (some say a matter of years), you will eventually find yourself needing to consider HL7 V3 processing in your healthcare integration plans. This appendix addresses the differences between HL7 V3 and HL7 V2.x and details a scenario that shows the integration of HL7 V3 applications with existing HL7 V2.x applications.

What is HL7 Version 3?

As discussed in Chapter 7, the 2.x versions of the HL7 standard have lost a significant amount of their original effectiveness over time because of the amount of optionality that is built into the standard. Further, the first 2.x versions of HL7 were created prior to the widespread adoption of XML. As the standard developed, the flat file, delimited data structure was kept because of backwards compatibility concerns. This means that the 2.x versions of HL7 do not contain syntactical rules, so you must look outside of the actual data (to the written standard) to determine if the message is constructed correctly.

Eventually, with the growing awareness of the benefits provided by XML, the fact that the 2.x versions of HL7 do not inherently contain information on both the message content and message structure has come to be seen as a limitation.

In its consideration of an updated version of the HL7 standard, the HL7 organization determined that XML encoding would provide the necessary groundwork for the much needed changes to the 2.x versions. Because it is so radically different from the 2.x versions, Version 3 constitutes the first real modeling effort by the HL7 organization.

In Version 3, HL7 data is encoded as XML and contains several layers of data modeling information before the actual message content. Figure B.1 below shows an example of an HL7 Version 3 message.

```
- <ns0:POLB_IN002121 xmlns:ns0="urn:hl7-org:v3">
    <ns0:creationTime value="2004-11-03T15:59:08" />
    <ns0:acceptAckCode code="AL" />
    <ns0:versionId>V3R1B6</ns0:versionId>
  - <ns0:controlActProcess>
    - <ns0:subject>
      - <ns0:ObservationOrder classCode="OBS" moodCoc
          type="Observation">
          <ns0:id root="2.16.840.1.113883.9876.349"
            extension="187963" />
          <ns0:effectiveTime value="200401291745" />
        - <ns0:recordTarget>
          - <ns0:patient>
            - <ns0:patientLivingSubject>
              - <ns0:Person classCode="PSN"
                  determinerCode="INSTANCE">
```

Figure B.1: Sample HL7 Version 3 (HL7 V3) Data.

The data modeling in Version 3 is achieved through the use of a Unified Modeling Language (UML) and serves to define the structural requirements of the message alongside of the actual message content. Since the new version was to be in XML and necessarily could not be backwards compatible, the HL7 organization took the opportunity to tighten up the standard. Thus, Version 3 contains rigid message structure rules that do not exist in the 2.x versions.

Basically, the HL7 organization's motivation to develop a new version centered on the need to build a higher quality standard and to overcome built-in limitations of the 2.x versions. However, because of the detailed new modeling approach and the fact that the standard is centered on a foundation of XML, Version 3 also makes it easier to introduce new material into the standard.

Contents of Version 3

A Version 3 HL7 message is more complex than a Version 2.x message. A Version 3 message requires the use of many models and specifications, which are defined below.

- **Information Models** — HL7 Version 3 is built around a Reference Information Model (RIM). The RIM expresses data structures used across HL7. The RIM is refined to meet the needs of particular domains through the development of Domain Information Models. A message or group of related messages can then be further refined by using a Refined Message Information Model to specialize the RIM.

- **Data Types** — Each piece of data contains one or more attributes that define the structure of that particular piece of data. As models are specialized, the assigned data type may be specialized as well.

- **Vocabulary** — Every message contains a vocabulary specification that indicates the coding systems and value sets used in the message. These give meaning to the code values that may are used in the message.

- **Message Specifications** — Drawn from a Refined Message Information Model, a Message Specification contains the attributes needed to support a specific trigger event. Unlike a model, a message specification is "serialized," which means it has a defined order for its contents. This allows messages to be parsed.

- **Conformance Profiles** — Published by a trading partner, a conformance profile specifies how a particular message specification is to be implemented in a particular situation. It resolves any remaining optionality in the message specification by indicating what particular code values are allowed and whether or not a particular attribute is to be valued.

Figure B.2 below shows the relationship between these Version 3 messaging components.

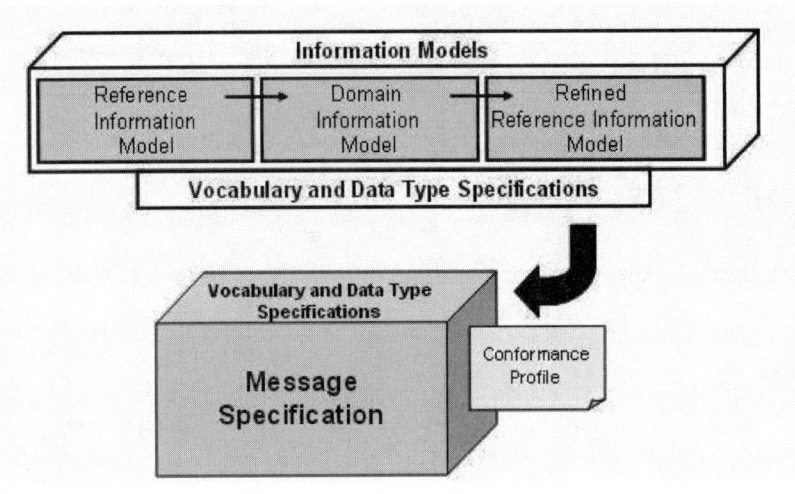

Figure B.2: HL7 V3 Messaging Components.

As you can see from the diagram, in Version 3, Information Models of increasing specification (shown from left to right in Figure B.2) are used to create a Message Specification for a particular type of Version 3 message, such as a Lab Result. Along the way, vocabulary and data type specifications are used to define the data that is used in the message. Finally, a conformance profile can also be used to further document the data values to be used in the message.

Once a message specification is finalized, an XSD schema is created to define the message type for that particular message specification. The fact that the message specification must contain vocabulary and data type specifications means that it takes multiple schemas to support the V3 message. In fact, it is not uncommon to have several different schemas used to define the message specification, and to also have separate schemas for the vocabulary and code sets.

For instance, the body of the message is considered the payload. You will most likely have a separate schema (called a Payload Schema) that defines the message body. Then, there are two other message parts involved, each defined by a separate schema: the transport wrapper and control event wrapper. Finally, there are schemas that define the data elements and coding involved in the structure: CMET schemas, data types schemas, and vocabulary schemas. In order to process a single Version 3 HL7 message, you will need to combine all of these separate schemas into a single customized one. Figure B.3 below shows a customized V3 HL7 message schema for an observation request message.

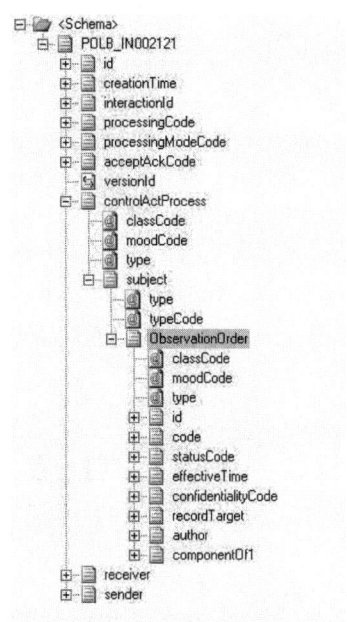

```
<Schema>
  POLB_IN002121
    id
    creationTime
    interactionId
    processingCode
    processingModeCode
    acceptAckCode
    versionId
    controlActProcess
      classCode
      moodCode
      type
      subject
        type
        typeCode
        ObservationOrder
          classCode
          moodCode
          type
          id
          code
          statusCode
          effectiveTime
          confidentialityCode
          recordTarget
          author
          componentOf1
    receiver
    sender
```

Figure B.3: HL7 V3 Message Schema for an Observation Request Message.

The Challenges of HL7 Version 3 Integration

Market realities dictate that Version 3 will need to co-exist with Version 2.x for quite some time. With over 90% of the hospitals in the United States and 27 countries worldwide currently utilizing HL7 V2.x message structures, the move to Version 3 will most likely be a slow and steady process at best. That means that the primary challenge of any Version 3 integration will be integrating the new standard with the established V2.x infrastructure within the enterprise.

Integration between different versions within the 2.x standard was facilitated by the backwards compatibility rules designed into the 2.x standard. However, because V3 is an XML format that has multiple encoding layers, by definition it is not backwards compatible with the flat file, non-XML format of the 2.x versions. To accomplish a nexus between the two standards requires an integration engine like BizTalk Server 2004, which is capable of understanding and processing both versions. In addition to being able to parse and validate both standards, the integration tool must provide the capability to map data elements between the two versions so that data can be seamlessly translated between formats.

In addition to translating data elements between versions, a complete Version 3 integration will require the enforcement of strict business rules. Because of the backwards compatibility rules inherent in the 2.x standard, the standard has been distilled down to essentially an agreed-upon framework for integration. Version 3 is much stricter than the 2.x standard. Version 3 incorporates more trigger events and message formats than the 2.x versions, with very little optionality.

BizTalk Server 2004 Meets the Challenge of V3 Integrations

Because HL7 V3 messages are encoded with XML, BizTalk provides support for Version 3 without the need for a special accelerator. The added benefit that BizTalk provides for HL7 V3 processing is that, beyond a basic ability to parse and validate the data, BizTalk brings with it a flexible and dynamic mapping tool that can be used to seamlessly translate data elements between standards, as well as enforce the data modeling requirements found in the V3 message specification. The strict business rules associated with V3 data creation can also be accommodated through BizTalk's orchestration and business rules engine.

Beyond its native support for HL7 V3, BizTalk can easily be extended to accommodate the challenges raised by interoperability between systems utilizing both the HL7 V2.x and V3 standards. As discussed in Chapter 8, the BizTalk Accelerator for HL7 enables BizTalk to parse and validate HL7 V2.x data as well as to seamlessly create data in the 2.x structure.

By utilizing the basic components of BizTalk together with the HL7 pipelines provided with the HL7 Accelerator, it is possible to design and implement a robust HL7 V3 integration. The next section defines how these BizTalk components could be designed and deployed in order to achieve basic integration between a system processing HL7 V3 order messages and an application utilizing an HL7 V2.4 ORM and ORU format.

Version 3 Integration Use Case: Establishing Interoperability between Version 3 and Version 2.4 Applications

Because HL7 V3 is so different from HL7 V2.x, a move to HL7 V3 is not likely to occur in a single enterprise across all of its applications at the same time. Rather, new applications will begin to utilize the V3 standard while older applications will continue to process only V2.x formats. Thus, the earliest type of integration scenario encountered will most likely be the requirement to design interoperability between V3 and V2.x applications.

The steps defined in the following sections address a common situation where a clinical information system communicates with a clinical laboratory. A typical scenario in that interface is one in which the clinical information system transmits an order to the laboratory, which performs a test, and responds with the results of the test.

The specific integration challenge to be addressed is the case in which the Lab has migrated to using HL7 Version 3, while the clinical information system is still using Version 2.4. The task at hand is to carry out two mappings:

- Accept the V2.4 ORM (order message) and transform it into a Version 3 Observation Request

- Accept a Version 3 Observation Event and transform it into a V2.4 ORU (order result)

Figure B.4 shows the message flow addressed by this integration use case.

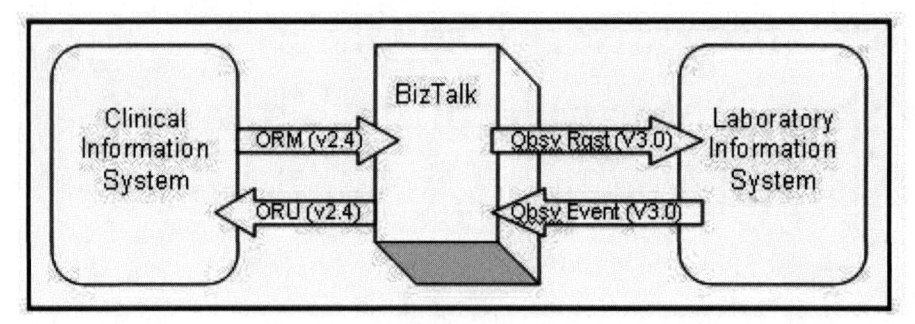

Figure B.4: Use Case Message Flow.

Integration Scenario One

This section addresses the first part of this common integration challenge through the creation of BizTalk components designed around receiving and processing an HL7 V2.4 ORM message into a V3 Laboratory Observation Request.

This scenario will require the following BizTalk components:

- The HL7 Accelerator (providing the necessary HL7 V2.4 schema and the HL7 Receive Pipeline to parse and validate the V2.4-formatted data into an XML format used internally by BizTalk)

- Version 3 message schema defining the Observation Request format

- A map translating the V2.4 data elements into the V3 format

Configuring the HL7 Accelerator to Process the V2.4 Message

To start our development process, we will focus on preparing BizTalk to correctly parse and validate the incoming V2.4 ORM^O01. The following steps are addressed in Chapter 8 at a high level and are detailed here for use in demonstrating the HL7 V3 to HL7 V2.x interoperability.

Once you have installed the HL7 Accelerator, you will have an HL7 Receive Pipeline already deployed into your configuration database. As shown in Figure B.5 below, this is the pipeline that you will use to configure the receive location that will receive the incoming message. The HL7 Receive Pipeline has an HL7 Disassembler component that will parse the incoming message from its flat file format into the XML format used internally by BizTalk.

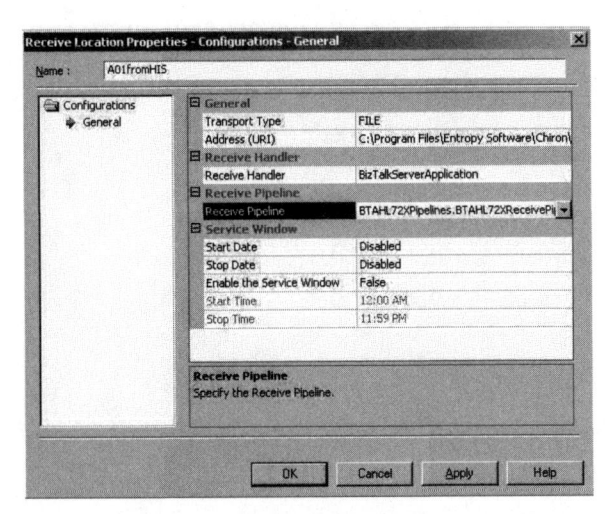

Figure B.5: Receive Location Using the HL7 Receive Pipeline.

Once the data is parsed, the HL7 Disassembler component will also validate the data against the V2.4 ORM^O01 schema provided by the Accelerator. This means that your first development step will be to deploy the V2.4 schema that will be used by the Accelerator when validating the message. Assuming that this is your initial development activity after installing the HL7 Accelerator, there are three different projects that you will need to deploy in order to correctly parse and validate your data:

- The BTAHL7V2XCommonProject
- The BTAHL7V24CommonProject
- The V2.4 HL7 ORM^O01 Schema

Deploy the MSH Segment Schema

The **MSH** Segment is used to identify the correct message body schema to use to validate the message. This schema must be deployed initially upon Accelerator installation, as it will be used for all of your V2.x processing. To deploy it, add a new project to your solution and choose **Add a New Item**. The MSH schema is contained in a project in the HL7 Projects category called BTAHL7V2XCommon Project (as shown in Figure B.6).

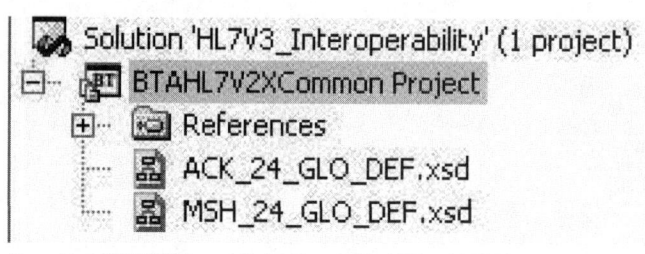

```
Solution 'HL7V3_Interoperability' (1 project)
  BTAHL7V2XCommon Project
    References
    ACK_24_GLO_DEF.xsd
    MSH_24_GLO_DEF.xsd
```

Figure B.6: BTAHL72XCommonProject Contains the MSH and ACK Schemas.

After creating and setting a required Assembly Key (.snk) file, deploy this project.

> **NOTE**
>
> This is a one-time step that is necessary for all of your HL7 processing because now the message header and acknowledgement schemas are available in the configuration database.

Deploy the V2.4 Dictionary Schema

Definitional schemas are provided for each of the 2.X versions in predefined BizTalk projects by version. You will need to deploy the appropriate project for the HL7 version you are processing. In the Solution Explorer, add a new HL7 project. The projects are located under HL7 schema projects; the one you need to add is called BTAHL7V24Common Project, where the "V24" indicates the version number. When this opens in the Solution Explorer, notice that three schemas—datatypes_231.xsd, segments_231.xsd, and tablevalues_231.xsd—are included in the project, as shown in Figure B.7.

Appendix B - HL7 Version 3 Processing with BizTalk Server 2004

```
BTAHL7V24Common Project
    References
    datatypes_24.xsd
    segments_24.xsd
    tablevalues_24.xsd
```

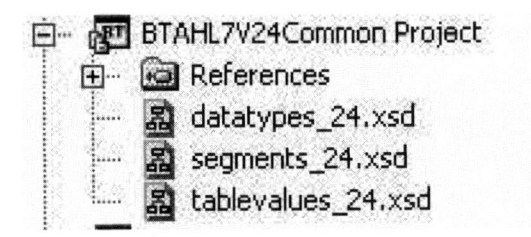

Figure B.7: BTAHL7V24CommonProject Contains the Definitional Schema for Use with All of the V2.4 HL7 Schemas.

After applying the necessary Assembly Key (.snk) file, deploy this project.

> **NOTE**
>
> This is a one-time step that is necessary for your entire Version 2.4 processing because now the definitional schemas referenced by all Version 2.4 schemas are available in the configuration database.

Deploy the V2.4 ORM^O01 Message Schema

Once the header and version-specific definitional schemas are deployed, you will configure and deploy message-specific schemas as necessary for your HL7 processing. In the Solution Explorer, add an empty HL7 project as a new project. In this project, you will add a reference to the previously deployed project containing the definitional schemas for the message version you are processing. For instance, since you are processing a Version 2.4 ORM message, you will reference the Version2.4CommonProject you just deployed, as seen in Figure B.8.

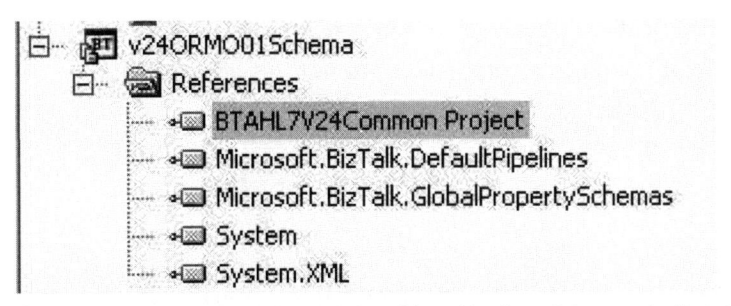

```
v24ORMO01Schema
    References
        BTAHL7V24Common Project
        Microsoft.BizTalk.DefaultPipelines
        Microsoft.BizTalk.GlobalPropertySchemas
        System
        System.XML
```

Figure B.8: The Project Containing the HL7 Message Schema Must Have a Reference to that Version's Common Project.

Once the reference is added, you will add a message schema to this project for each message type you are processing:

1. Add a new item to the project, selecting **BTAHL7Schemas** under **BizTalk Project Items** in the category pane of the **Add New Item** dialog box.

2. In the **HL7 Schema Selector** dialog box, select the version and message type you are interested in. Since you are processing a Version 2.4 ORM^O01 message, select 2.4 for the **Version**, ORM for **Message Type**, and 001 for the **Event Type**, then click the **Finish** button (see Figure B.9). This will add the message definition schema to your project.

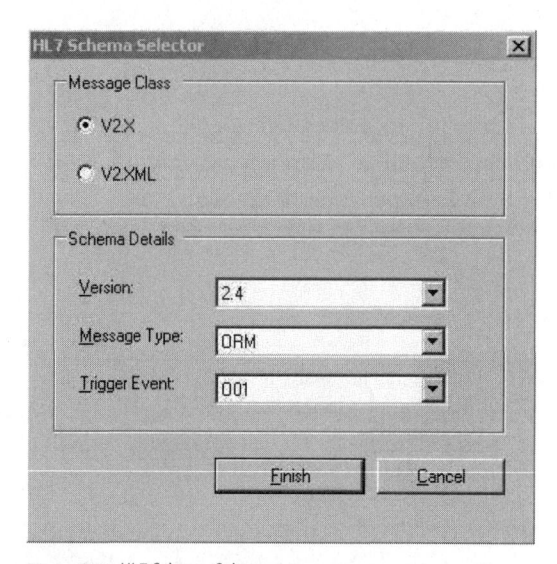

Figure B.9: HL7 Schema Selector.

3. The **HL7 Schema Selector** dialog box will remain open for you to add other schemas into this project. Since we will be processing a V2.4 ORU^R01 message in Integration Scenario Two that follows this section, repeat the selection steps to add a V2.4 ORU R01 schema to the project. Once complete, click the **Cancel** button to close the dialog box.

4. Once you have added a message schema for each message type that you are processing, apply the necessary Assembly Key (.snk) file and deploy this project. Once done, these are the schemas you will reference and use in your V2.4 maps and orchestrations.

Configuring BizTalk to Process the V3 Outgoing Message

Because HL7 V3 is encoded as XML, you do not need the HL7 Accelerator to process V3 messages. Rather, you will need to simply add an XSD schema for the message type you desire to a BizTalk project and then deploy it.

The V3 standard is really a body of standards, some of which are still being finalized. Thus, to use "official" schemas, you should use "balloted" schemas—those which have been finalized under the HL7 organization's processes. To access balloted schemas, visit http://www.hl7.org/v3ballot/html/index.htm.

Once you have downloaded your desired schemas, you will want to combine them into a single schema and customize them as necessary using referencing, etc. For that reason, there is no single "official" V3 schema.

In the next step, you will use a BizTalk map to translate the V2.4 data into the V3 message format. Maps require you to declare both a source and destination schema. You will need use the V3 schema for the ORM message as your destination schema. To accomplish this task, you will need to first deploy the V3 ORM schema.

Deploy the V3 Message Schema

To deploy the schema, add a new project to your solution. Choose **Add an Existing Item** and add the V3 XSD schema for the V3 Observation Request message type. After applying the necessary Assembly Key (.snk) file, deploy this project.

Configure and Deploy a Map Creating the V3 Message Structure

Now that you have deployed your source and target schemas, you are ready to create a map, according to the following steps:

1. To create a BizTalk map, you will add a new project to your solution to hold your map and name it according to what the map is accomplishing, such as `V24ORM_to_V3ObsvReqst`.

2. Add references to the projects containing your V2.4 definitional and structure schemas, as well as to your V3 message schemas.

3. Add a BizTalk Map as a new item into this project. You should name the map the same as the project name, such as `V240RM_to_V3ObsvReqst.btm` in this example.

4. Define your source and destination schemas. The source schema will be the V2.4 message schema project and the destination schema will be the V3 message schema project.

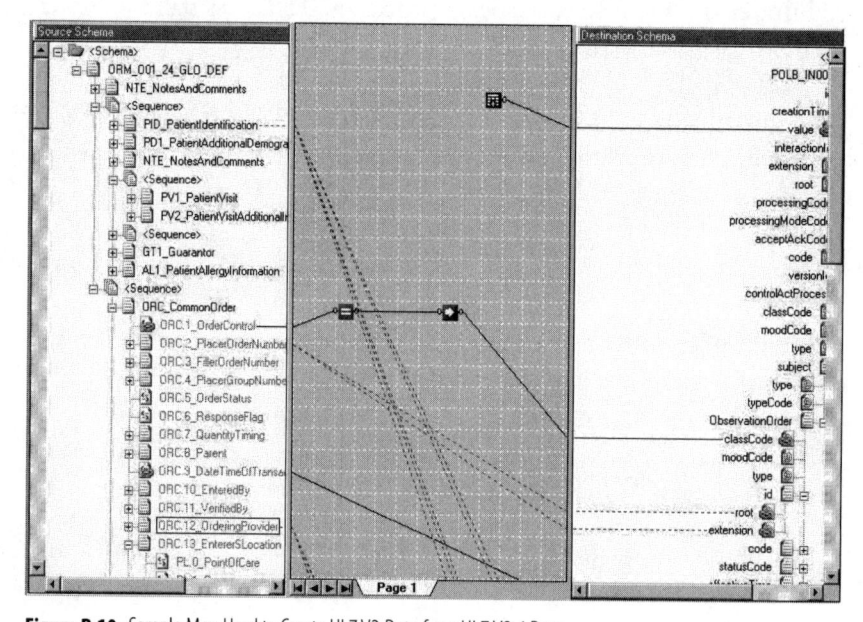

Figure B.10: Sample Map Used to Create HL7 V3 Data from HL7 V2.4 Data.

Figure B.10 shows a map that can be used to create a V3 Observation Request from a V2.4 ORM. The map is only a small sampling of the actual mapping that would need to be performed to completely create the V3 data structure from a V2.4 ORM.

5. To fully configure your map, you will locate the incoming data fields in the V2.4 message and drag and drop them into the proper location in the V3 message structure. Because of the strict coding and structure rules of the V3 format, some of your map rules will require hard coding of values, while others will require you to evaluate the incoming field for a certain value before you conditionally create an outgoing value. To hard code a

value, access the **Properties** window for the element and enter the desired text into the **Value** row in the **Properties** window. To evaluate incoming data to conditionally create output data, you will use a combination of a logical functoid and a value mapping functoid.

Basically, with the exception of the simplest maps, you will use functions such as logical evaluation and value mapping, string manipulation, database access, and others to create the required V3 structure. These functions, called *functoids* in BizTalk, can be found in the toolbox and inserted into the map grid between the source and target panes.

> **NOTE**
>
> Functoids can be chained so that the output of one functoid can be the input to another. If you cannot locate a functoid that meets your specific needs, you can always utilize the script functoid. The script functoid is an open-ended functoid that will allow you to write in-line code in C#, Visual Basic .NET, J# or even XSLT. Script functoids can also call code from referenced assemblies.

When complete, test the map to ensure that your map rules executed in the manner intended. Once you are satisfied with the map output, you will add the necessary Assembly Key (.snk) file and deploy the map project. Once deployed, refresh the configuration database to ensure your access to the maps in the next configuration steps.

Configure BizTalk to Call the V2.4 to V3 Map

Once you have deployed a map, it can be called in several different ways:

- Being bound to a receive port
- Being bound to a send port
- From an orchestration through the Transform shape

The simplest way to run a map is to bind it to either a send or receive port. If your integration scenario or business process has no orchestration defined for it, bind your map to either a send or receive port.

As discussed in Chapter 4, if you choose to bind a map to the receive port, messages will be stored in the message box as the *output* format of the map. Therefore, any targets subscribing to that message will pick up the output of the map, not the original sending system's format. Use this approach when most targets require the message to be translated or enriched in the same way before it can be processed. This results in the logic only being executed once on the receive side, instead of once for each target.

When a map is bound to a send port, only the target for that specific port will receive the output of the map. No other targets will receive that output unless their send port is configured to call the same map (resulting in the map being called once for each send port bound to it). Bind a map to a send port when you wish to perform target-specific transformation, translation, or enrichment.

Bind a map to an orchestration when orchestration-specific transformation, translation, or enrichment needs to be performed or when multiple maps need to be called in a single subscription.

In the scenario, we are processing from a single V2.4 application to a single V3 application. Because the transformation is target-specific, we will call the map by binding it to the send port. To accomplish this, when configuring your send port, select **Outbound Maps** under **Filters & Maps** in the left navigation screen. On the right side of the dialog box, select the map that you wish to apply to this send port.

In addition to calling the map, you will configure the send port to use the XMLTransport pipeline provided with BizTalk, add a subscription, then enlist and start the send port.

You are now ready to test the scenario. To do this, place a sample V2.4 file into the receive location you configured. You should see a V3 formatted message appear in the file location specified in your send port.

Integration Scenario Two

Building on the premise that earliest type of integration scenario encountered will most likely be the requirement to design interoperability between V3 and V2.x applications, this section addresses the need to receive and process a V3 Result Event message into a V2.4 ORU message format.

This scenario will require the following BizTalk components:

- Version 3 message schema defining the Observation Result Event format (Deployed similarly to the schema from Integration Scenario One)

- A map translating the V3 data elements into the V2.4 format

- An orchestration used to build the V2.4 **MSH** Segment onto the V2.4 message body created by the V3 to V2.4 map

- The HL7 Accelerator (providing the necessary HL7 V2.4 schema and the HL7 Send Pipeline to serialize the V2.4-formatted data from BizTalk's internal XML format to the V2.4 flat file format)

Configuring BizTalk to Process the V3 Incoming Message

As discussed earlier, you do not need the HL7 Accelerator to process V3 messages. To receive and process V3 messages, you will use the default XML Receive Pipeline. To send the data to a map or an orchestration, you will also need to deploy the appropriate V3 message schema.

Deploy the V3 Message Schema

As with Integration Scenario One, you will need to deploy a schema that defines the V3 message that you are processing. In this case, we are receiving a V3 Observation Event. Once we have downloaded all of the necessary schemas to support our V3 message from the HL7 website and customized them as desired, we will add this to our project as an existing item. Then, we will build and deploy the project (or redeploy if placing it in an already deployed project).

Configure a Map to Translate the V3 Data Elements into the V2.4 Format

In order to create the V2.4 message body structure that you desire, you will create, configure, and deploy a map in a similar fashion to what was described in Integration Scenario One. However, in this case, the source schema will be the V3 message schema and the destination schema will be the V2.4 message schema. As with the previously described map, you will need to add references into the map project for both schemas as well as for the V2.4 dictionary schema.

The mapping steps necessary to create a V2.4 structure are not as complex as those needed to create a V3 structure, because the V2.x standard is simpler than the V3 standard. Most commonly, when mapping V3 data into a V2.x format, the majority of your mapping will involve dragging and dropping incoming elements into the desired output location.

When complete, you will want to test the map to ensure that your map rules executed in the manner intended. Once you are satisfied with the map output, you will add the necessary Assembly Key (.snk) file and deploy the map project. Once deployed, you will want to refresh the configuration database to ensure your access to the maps in the next configuration steps.

In the previous section, we called the map used to create our outbound V3 structure by binding it to a send port. However, when creating V2.x structures, we will not be able to fully create the message structure in this manner. Due to the way the HL7 Accelerator handles V2.x messages, we will need to call this map in an orchestration so that we can add the **MSH** Segment to the top of the message body created by the map.

Creating a Complete V2.4 Message Through an Orchestration

As discussed in Chapter 8, the V2.x message schemas do not contain the **MSH** Segment, because that segment is parsed differently by the HL7 Accelerator. The HL7 Accelerator treats the V2.x message structure as three distinct units: the message header (**MSH** Segment), the message body (all standard-defined segments after the **MSH** Segment), and Z-segments. The impact of this is that when using a map to create a V2.x HL7 message structure, you will need to use an orchestration to assign the various message structure parts into a single structure for outbound processing through the HL7 Send Pipeline. You must use the HL7 Send Pipeline when sending HL7 V2.x data outbound from BizTalk, because it contains the HL7 Assembler, which serializes the data from BizTalk's internal XML structure into the flat file 2.x structure.

To configure an orchestration to assign the three parts of a V2.4 structure into a single unit, you will need to add a new project to your Solution, and add an orchestration as a new item into the project. Once this is complete, add references to the V3 and V2.4 message schema (including the V2.4 dictionary schema) as well as to the V3ObsvEvent_ to_V24ORU map. You will also need to add a reference to the Microsoft.Solutions. BTAHL7Schemas.dll that is located in <HL7 Accelerator install directory>\Program Files\Microsoft BizTalk Accelerator for HL7 1.0\Bin.

Because orchestrations are used to configure business processes, there are many required configuration steps in designing an orchestration. The following procedure lists the steps necessary to receive a V3 message into an orchestration, call a map to transform the V3 data into a V2.4 message structure, assign an **MSH** Segment to the V2.4 Message Body, and send the completed, unified V2.4 message from the orchestration. Once it leaves the orchestration, the V2.4 message will be routed through a send port using the HL7 Send Pipeline so that the data that leaves BizTalk will be a V2.4-formatted flat file.

Configuring an Orchestration

The following procedure details the steps necessary to configure an orchestration to create a complete HL7 message.

1. Add a **Receive** shape to the orchestration. Name it `Receive_V3ObsvEvent` and set the **Activate** property to **True**.

2. Add a **Transform** shape under the **Receive** shape. Name the **Construct** shape `ConstructV24ORUbody` and name the **Transform** shape `V2.4ORU_Body_Creation`.

3. Add a **Message Assignment** shape under the **ConstructV24ORUbody Construct Message** shape. Name the **Construct** shape `Construct Final ORU` and name the **Assignment** shape `V24ORU_Final_Construct`.

4. Add a **Send** shape under the **V24ORU_Final_Construct** shape. Name it `SendV24ORU`.

5. In the **Orchestration View** window, add the message definitions you need:

    - **V3ObsEvent** = V3ObsvEvent.xsd

    - **V24ORUbody** = ORU_R01_24_GLO_DEF.xsd

    - **finalV24ORUmessage** = to be configured below

6. In the **Orchestration View** window, move under **Types** and add a **Multi-Part Message Type** called **final V24ORUmessageType**. Expand the entry and change the **Identifier** on **MessagePart_1** to `BodySegments`. Then, add two more message parts called **MSHSegment** and **ZSegment**.

7. In the **Properties** window for **BodySegments**, under **Type**, select **Schemas**, **<Select from referenced assembly>** to select the ORU_R01_24_GLO_DEF.xsd.

8. In the **Properties** window for **MSHSegment**, under **Type**, select **.NET Classes**, and then click **<Select from referenced assemblies>**. In the **Select Artifact Type** dialog box, in the left pane, click **System.Xml**. In the right pane, click **XmlDocument**, and then click the **OK** button.

9. In the **Properties** window for **ZSegment**, under **Type**, select **.NET Classes**, then select **System.String** from the list.

10. Move to the **Messages** entry, select **finalV24ORMO01message** and open its **Properties** window. Click **Message Type**, expand **Multi-part Message Types**, and then click **<ProjectName>. final V24ORUmessageType**.

11. In the **Orchestration View** window, right-click **Variables**, and then click **New Variable** to create **Variable_1**. In the **Properties** pane for **Variable_1**, click **Identifier**, and type the new name `HeaderInfo`. Click **Type**, and then double-click **<.NET Class>**. In the left pane of the **Select Artifact** window, click **System.Xml**; in the right pane, click **XmlDocument**, and then click the **OK** button.

12. To configure your orchestration shapes, assign the following messages to the appropriate shape:

    - **Receive** = ObsEvent
    - **ContructV24ORUbody** = V24ORUbody
    - **ConstructFinalORU** = finalV24ORUmessage
    - **SendV24ORU** = finalV24ORUmessage

13. In the **Properties** window for the **Transform** shape, call the V3ObsvEvent_to_V24ORU map.

    - The Source Variable = V3ObsEvent
    - The Destination Variable = V24ORUbody

14. To configure the **ConstructFinalORU** shape, move into its **Properties** window and select **Messages Constructed**, and then select the **finalV24ORUmessage** check box in the drop-down list.

15. To configure the **V24ORU_Final_Construct** Assignment shape, go to its **Properties** window, click **Expression**, and then click the ellipsis (…) button to open BizTalk Expression Editor. Type the code in Listing B.1 into the Expression shape, and then click the **OK** button.

```
HeaderInfo = new System.Xml.XmlDocument();
↪HeaderInfo.LoadXml("<ns0:MSH_24_GLO_DEF xmlns:ns0=\"http://microsoft.
↪com/HealthCare/HL7/2X\"><MSH><MSH.2_EncodingCharacters>^~\\&amp;</MSH.2_E
↪ncodingCharacters><MSH.3_SendingApplication><HD.0_NamespaceId>SrcApp</
↪HD.0_NamespaceId><HD.1_UniversalId>SrcAppUid</HD.1_UniversalId></
↪MSH.3_SendingApplication><MSH.4_SendingFacility><HD.0_NamespaceId>srcFac</
↪HD.0_NamespaceId><HD.1_UniversalId>srcFacUid</HD.1_UniversalId></MSH.4_
↪SendingFacility><MSH.5_ReceivingApplication><HD.0_NamespaceId>dstApp</
↪HD.0_NamespaceId><HD.1_UniversalId>dstAppUid</HD.1_UniversalId></MSH.5_R
↪eceivingApplication><MSH.6_ReceivingFacility><HD.0_NamespaceId>dstFac</
↪HD.0_NamespaceId><HD.1_UniversalId>dstFacUid</HD.1_UniversalId></
↪MSH.6_ReceivingFacility><MSH.7_DateTimeOfMessage><TS.1>200307092343</
↪TS.1></MSH.7_DateTimeOfMessage><MSH.8_Security>sec</MSH.8_Security><MSH.9_
↪MessageType><CM_MSG.0_MessageType>ORU</CM_MSG.0_MessageType><CM_MSG.1_
↪TriggerEvent>R01</CM_MSG.1_TriggerEvent></MSH.9_MessageType><MSH.10_Messa
↪geControlId>msgid2134</MSH.10_MessageControlId><MSH.11_ProcessingId><PT.0_
↪ProcessingId>P</PT.0_ProcessingId></MSH.11_ProcessingId><MSH.12_
↪VersionId><VID.0_VersionId>2.4</VID.0_VersionId></MSH.12_VersionId></
↪MSH></ns0:MSH_24_GLO_DEF>");

finalv24ORUmessage.MSHSegment = HeaderInfo;
finalv24ORUmessage.BodySegments = v24ORUbody;
finalv24ORUmessage.ZSegment = "";

finalv24ORUmessage(BTAHL7Schemas.MSH1) = 124;
finalv24ORUmessage(BTAHL7Schemas.MSH2) = "^~\\&";
finalv24ORUmessage(BTAHL7Schemas.ParseError) = false;
finalv24ORUmessage(BTAHL7Schemas.ZPartPresent) = false;

finalv24ORUmessage(BTAHL7Schemas.SegmentDelimiter2Char) = true;
```

Listing B.1: Expression Code.

> **🏷️ BONUS**
>
> This code is contained in a file called Orchestration Expression.txt, available as a free download when you register this book at www.agilitypress.com.

> **✒️ NOTE**
>
> The first block of the expression text is an example hard-coded XML header. The BTAHL7 serializer requires a header segment. You can customize these header values according to the needs of your environment. The second block of the preceding text defines the three message parts required in a multi-part message. BTAHL7 serializer requires a multi-part message. The third block of the preceding text contains the promoted properties that the BTAHL7 serializer examines in order to correctly serialize an XML message into an HL7 flat-file message.

16. Create the necessary ports for the orchestration.

When complete, your orchestration should look like Figure B.11 below.

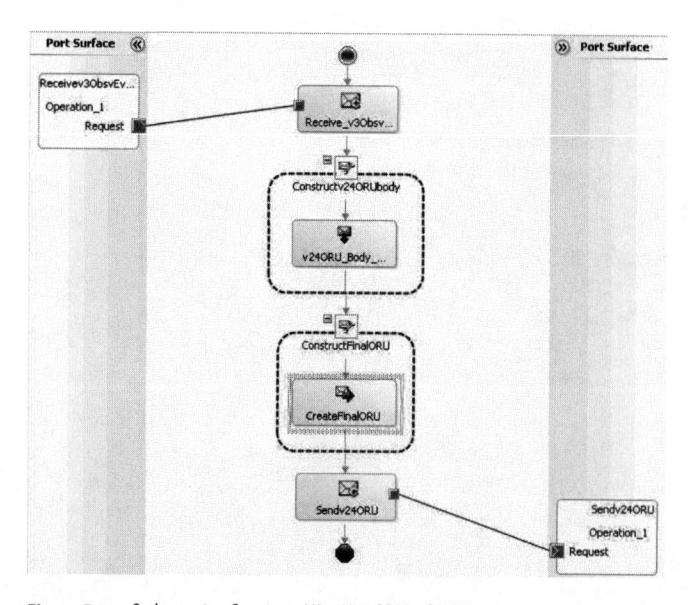

Figure B.11: Orchestration Creating a V2.4 HL7 ORM^001 Message.

Once the orchestration is fully configured, you will add the necessary Assembly key (.snk) file, build and deploy it. You will need to refresh the configuration database to have access to the orchestration in BizTalk Explorer.

Once you have configured your physical send port in the next step, you will bind this orchestration to that send port as well as to a V3 receive location created to receive the V3 Observation Event file. Once bound, you will enlist and start the orchestration in order to test the scenario.

Testing the Scenario

This scenario, like the previous one, depends on the proper configuration of the HL7 Accelerator. However, assuming that the necessary V2.4 schemas remain deployed from the previous scenario, you do not need to take any further action to configure the HL7 Accelerator. Rather, the only step you will need to complete is to configure a send port to use the HL7 Send Pipeline provided by the HL7 Accelerator.

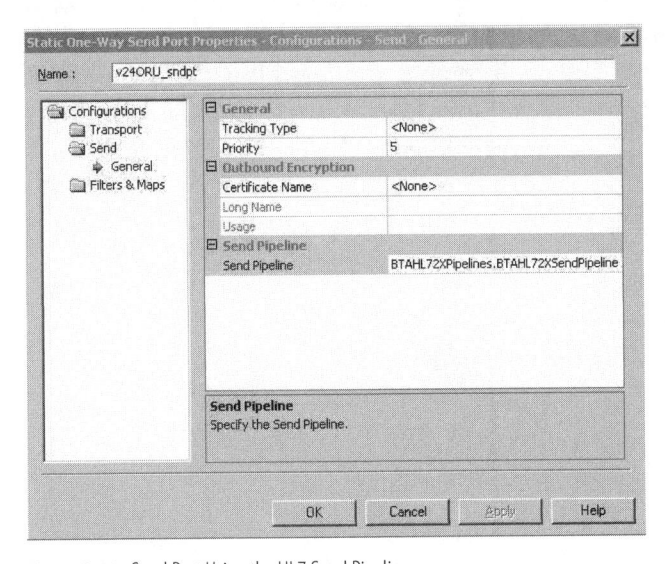

Figure B.12: Send Port Using the HL7 Send Pipeline.

As seen in Figure B.12, in order to configure a send port to serialize HL7 data correctly, you simply need to configure it to use the HL7 Send Pipeline. You do not need to place a filter on the port, as the V3_to_V24_ORM_Orchestration will be bound to the port.

As the orchestration is enlisted, you will enable, enlist, and start your receive and send ports. Then, to test the scenario, you simply place V3 sample data in your receive location, then move to your send port location and view the created V2.4 file.

Summary

These two processing scenarios were chosen because their simplicity can be used as a foundation for more complex processing needs. Since it is estimated that the majority of HL7 V3 processing will involve interfacing with V2.x message formats, these two scenarios demonstrate how the flexibility of BizTalk Server 2004 makes it an ideal solution for all of your HL7 processing needs.

As HL7 V3 evolves and is finalized as a standard, the schema needs for defining it may become more complex. Regardless of how HL7 V3 evolves, its fundamental XML formatting means that BizTalk Server 2004 will be able to process it without the aid of an additional accelerator. However, to achieve interoperability between V3 and V2.x systems, you will need the added components provided by the HL7 Accelerator.

For more information on the evolving V3 HL7 standard, visit www.HL7.org.

Glossary

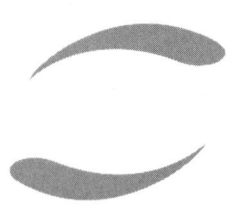

Adapter	A pre-built set of logic that enables a "dial-tone" connection to an application's API, or a technical protocol, such as ODBC, or HTTP. Adapters shield the developer from the technical underpinnings of an API or protocol.
Business Process Integration (BPI)	Next-generation of enterprise application integration, which enables a business-level view of how to build, define, and manage how disparate systems work together in a specific business context. BizTalk Server 2004 is a platform for business process integration.
Business Process Management (BPM)	A complementary technology to a business process integration platform focused on enabling the enterprise business process by managing how people interact with a business process.
Business Activity Monitoring (BAM)	A platform that enables real-time visibility into a business process, often implemented in conjunction with a BPM or BPI platform.
Electronic Data Interchange (EDI)	Electronic sharing of data between business entities according to a specific set of rules governing how the information will be packaged.
Enterprise Application Integration (EAI)	A collection of technologies that are collectively used to define and manage how to connect disparate applications within an enterprise.

Enterprise Business Process	An end-to-end definition of a how an enterprise handles a part of its business. Usually composed of integration scenarios, applications, and people.
Enterprise Service Bus (ESB)	An emerging technology that is a standards-based, messaging-oriented approach for building a service-oriented architecture.
Extensible Markup Language (XML)	A simple, very flexible text format that can be used to build documents that are easily interpreted by disparate systems.
HIPAA	Health Insurance Portability and Accountability Act of 1996. A United States federal law that, among other things, mandates the electronic transmission of healthcare data, establishes privacy interests in health information, and outlines strict security measures for protecting private healthcare information.
HL7 (Health Level Seven)	Data standard used to achieve interoperability between applications in a clinical healthcare environment. It also is the name of the volunteer organization charged with the creation of the data and interoperability standards.
Integration Broker	An EAI-focused product that acts as a messaging hub for the integration of applications.
Integration Pattern	A repeatable technique that can be applied to commonly encountered problems when building an interface.
Integration Scenario	A collection of integration patterns that solve a specific business problem.
Map	A definition of how systems with different message formats can communicate with each other. BizTalk maps are based on the XML Stylesheet – Transformation (XSLT) specification.
Orchestration	A state engine that can be used to correlate multiple messages, services, and actions (such as a map) together under one executable business process.
Payer	A healthcare entity that pays for healthcare services, such as an insurance company or third-party insurance administrator.

Pipeline	A software infrastructure that provides a series of discrete stages for processing inbound and outbound messages, running them in a defined order to accomplish a task. Pipelines focus on the technical steps required to process a message, while orchestration is focused on the higher-level actions required to integrate a business process.
Provider	A clinical healthcare facility that provides health services, such as a hospital, clinic, or physician's office.
Service	A software component that performs work on behalf of another. A web service is a type of service that leverages SOAP, XML, and other related standards.
Service-Oriented Architecture	An enterprise architecture that is composed of a collection of services that are tied together using a consistent set of integration patterns.
Simple Object Access Protocol (SOAP)	Protocol used for web services that can employ many different transports, such as HTTP or messaging.
Web Services Description Language (WSDL)	A standards-based definition of the services offered by a SOAP-based web service.
XML Schema Definition (XSD)	The metadata definition for a valid XML document.

Further Resources

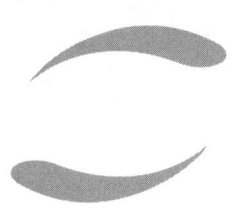

The resources listed in this section provide additional information on the topics covered in this book.

Architecture and Strategy

Beck, K. *Extreme Programming Explained*. Boston, MA: Addison-Wesley, 2000.

> *XP is a powerful methodology that is a good fit for many integration projects. If you are looking for a way to get projects done when specifications are unclear, this book is for you.*

Hohmann, L. *Beyond Software Architecture*. Boston, MA: Addison-Wesley, 2003.

> *A wonderful book on the business of software and the ingredients that go into successful solutions. The focus of this book is more oriented towards software vendors, but has many valuable insights for anyone involved in software architecture.*

Watts, D. *Six Degrees: The Science of a Connected Age*. New York: Norton, 2002.

> *A look at the interconnectedness of everything.*

BizTalk-Specific Resources

Woodgate, S. http://blogs.msdn.com/scottwoo

>   Scott Woodgate, the Product Manager for BTS04, has a very active blog covering many implementation questions and links to other good BTS resources.

Woodgate, S., Mohr, S., Loesgen, B. *Microsoft BizTalk Server 2004 Unleashed*. Indianapolis: Sams, 2004

>   A thorough developer's guide on how to use all of the features of BizTalk Server 2004.

http://www.gotdotnet.com

>   The .NET Framework community website. A great resource for all things .NET, including whitepapers, blogs, samples, and other downloads. Provides access to BizTalk Server 2004 newsgroups and updates.

http://www.microsoft.com/biztalk

>   Official Microsoft website for BizTalk Server 2004. Provides access to BizTalk resources, downloads, and whitepapers, and demos. Also provides access to information on the BizTalk Accelerator for HL7 and BizTalk Accelerator for HIPAA 3.0.

Business Resources

Murphy, T. *Achieving Business Value from Technology.* New York: John Wiley & Sons, 2002.

>   Analysis of how software projects can be measured and evaluated in business terms using Gartner's methodology.

General Technology

Developing XML Web Services and Server Components. Redmond, WA: Microsoft Press, 2003.

> *Part of the .NET Core training materials. This book is a good reference for how to develop web services using C# and VB .NET. A key thing to know when building service-oriented applications.*

Holzner, S. *Microsoft Visual C# .NET 2003 Kick Start*. Indianapolis: Sams, 2004.

> *A concise and clear reference for experienced programmers looking to get started quickly on learning C#.*

Healthcare Resources

http://www.hl7.org

> *Official website of the HL7 organization. A great place to access the HL7 data standards, whitepapers, articles, and other resources related to the interoperability of healthcare systems and clinical data management.*

http://www.HIMSS.org

> *Official website of the Healthcare Information and Management Systems Society (HIMSS). HIMSS is focused on providing leadership for the optimal use of healthcare information technology and management systems for the betterment of human health. This site offers access to articles and resources concerning the development of information technology in healthcare.*

http://www.cms.hhs.gov/hipaa

> *The HIPAA site for the Centers for Medicare & Medicaid Services. Features information about the health insurance reform and administrative simplification legislation.*

IMPORTANT NOTICE
REGISTER YOUR BOOK

Bonus Materials

Your book refers to valuable material that complements your learning experience. In order to download these materials you will need to register your book at http://www.agilitypress.com.

This bonus material is available after registration:

- ▶ Payer Implementation Example
- ▶ Provider Implementation Example

Registering your book

To register your book, follow these 7 easy steps:

1. Point your browser to:

   http://www.agilitypress.com.

2. Create an account and login.
3. Click the **My Books** link.
4. Click the **Register New Book** button.
5. Enter the registration number found on the back of the book (see Figure A).
6. Confirm registration and view your new book on the virtual bookshelf.
7. Click the spine of the desired book to view the available downloads and resources for the selected book.

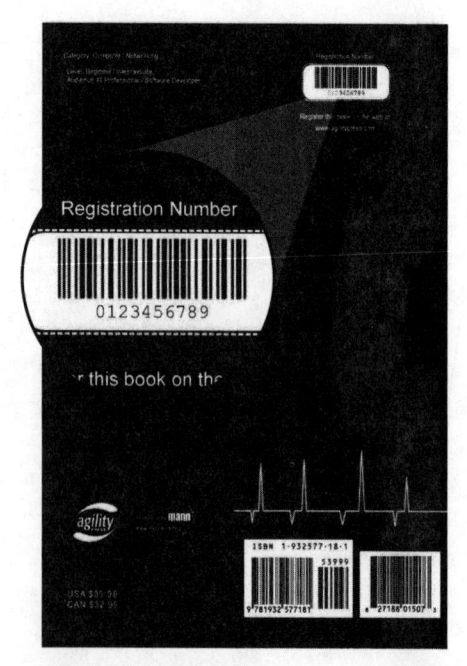

Figure A: Back of your book.